More praise for
The Miracle of Magnesium

"Every doctor and patient should read this comprehensive book on the many roles of magnesium. . . . I loved this book. Clearly written and packed with information, it offers a compendium on natural medicine and is an invaluable resource for both practitioner and public alike. It is the most comprehensive and well-referenced guide to the myriad benefits of magnesium published to date."
—Dr. Carolyn DeMarco
Author of *Take Charge of Your Body:
Women's Health Advisor*

"Throughout this volume and with utmost clarity, Carolyn Dean presents invaluable recommendations— based on the latest magnesium research. Virtually every American can benefit."
—Paul Pitchford
Author of *Healing with Whole Foods:
Asian Traditions and Modern Nutrition*

"Physicians and therapists have paid scant attention to this very important element, which is also involved in maintaining our good health. The massive evidence is here in this important book on magnesium. I am pleased to have been taking magnesium for so many years."
—Abram Hoffer, M.D.
Author of *Putting It All Together:
The New Orthomolecular Nutrition*

The Miracle of Magnesium

CAROLYN DEAN, M.D., N.D.

BALLANTINE BOOKS

NEW YORK

A Ballantine Book
Published by The Random House Publishing Group
Copyright © 2003 by Carolyn Dean, M.D., N.D.
Foreword copyright © 2003 by Dr. Bella Altura and Dr. Burton Altura

www.ballantinebooks.com

Library of Congress Cataloging-in-Publication Data

Dean, Carolyn.
The miracle of magnesium / Carolyn Dean.— 1st ed.
p.   cm.
Includes bibliographical references and index.
ISBN 0-345-44588-0
1. Magnesium deficiency diseases.   2. Magnesium—Health aspects.
I. Title.

RC627.M3 D43 2003
616.3'96—dc21
2002028159

Book design by Holly Johnson
Cover design by Mike Stromberg

Manufactured in the United States of America

First Edition: January 2003

5   7   9   10   8   6   4

To the Miracle Women in my life.
My mum, Rena, my three sisters: Chris (who
labored with me on the first drafts of "the wee maggie"),
Anne, and Evelyn. And my agent, Beth.
Thank you all.

Contents

Contents

Foreword

"Clearly there is more to life than magnesium" is one of the remarks from Dr. Dean's remarkable, almost encyclopedic, but very readable book. Her book is long overdue, for it gives the lay reader a chance to discover for him- or herself the many needs for this mineral in a healthy diet, and the reasons why this has not been emphasized in the everyday literature.

The requirements for magnesium in our diet is indeed a much neglected topic and this book by Dr. Dean brings the message home by her carefully written repetitive emphasis on the subject. That does not mean that there are not many other nutrients necessary in our daily food intake, as stated above, but the point she so clearly makes is that the public in general has not been notified to look for the proper amount of this mineral in the daily diet and of the many reasons magnesium is needed in our bodies.

After a cursory overview of the material, the book should be read as one would read an encyclopedia, that is pick out the parts one is particularly interested in, and then go back and try to read it all. This way the reader will get the gist of how important magnesium really is and how little he or she has been informed, be it from newspapers, magazines, or the rest of the news media. As the old adage says, "An ounce of prevention is worth its weight in gold," and so it is with a balanced nutrition, which includes this all-important mineral in adequate amounts.

(As to the other interesting parts of the book, our qualifications only allow us to comment on the material pertaining to the scientific basis for the need of magnesium.)

Dr. Bella T. Altura
Research Professor of
Physiology and Pharmacology
SUNY Downstate Medical Center
Brooklyn, New York

Dr. Burton M. Altura
Professor of Physiology,
Pharmacology, and Medicine
SUNY Downstate Medical Center
Brooklyn, New York

Introduction

From the 74th Congress, 2nd session, Senate Document no. 264:

> Do you know that most of us today are suffering from certain dangerous diet deficiencies which cannot be remedied until depleted soils from which our food comes are brought into proper mineral balance? The alarming fact is that foods (fruits, vegetables and grains) now being raised on millions of acres of land that no longer contain enough of certain minerals are starving us—no matter how much of them we eat. The truth is that our foods vary enormously in value, and some of them aren't worth eating as food. Our physical well-being is more directly dependent upon the minerals we take into our

systems than upon calories or vitamins or upon the precise proportions of starch, protein or carbohydrates we consume. Laboratory tests prove that the fruits, the vegetables, the grains, the eggs, and even the milk and the meats of today are not what they were a few generations ago. No man today can eat enough fruits and vegetables to supply his stomach with the mineral salts he requires for perfect health, because his stomach isn't big enough to hold them! And we are turning into a nation of big stomachs.

Do you know when those words were spoken in testimony before the Senate? Nineteen thirty-six! Today farmlands are even more mineral-deficient and fertilizers still don't fully replace those minerals. Magnesium is one of the most depleted minerals, yet one of the most important. We imagine that medicine has advanced to the stage of miracle cures, yet it's not technology that we're lacking but basic nutrients that power our bodies and give us our health.

Quick-fix medical solutions from doctors are all around us via television, the Internet, radio, and infomercials. In a world of rapid change, our bodies are going through peaks and crashes every day. We rely on double cappuccinos in the morning, a Power Bar for lunch, and an acupuncture treatment after work before we go to the gym for our energy hits. Harnessed to our cell phone, laptop, Palm Pilot, and pager, we're exhausting our natural physical stores of energy, straining our bodies' capacity to function and heal. Although we can't change our digital environment, we can learn how to preserve and rebuild our energy levels naturally.

Magnesium regulates more than 325 enzymes in the body, the most important of which produce, transport, store, and utilize energy. Many aspects of cell metabolism are regulated by magnesium, such as DNA and RNA synthesis, cell growth, and cell reproduction. Magnesium also orchestrates the electric current that sparks through the miles of nerves in our body. Magnesium has numerous physiological roles, among which are control of nerve action, the activity of the heart, neuromuscular transmission, muscular contraction, vascular tone, blood pressure, and peripheral blood flow. Magnesium modulates and controls the entry and release of calcium from the cell, which determines muscular activity. Without magnesium, muscle and nerve functions are compromised and energy is diminished. We are operating with the power turned off. Muscular weakness, soft bones, anxiety, heart attacks, arrhythmia, and even seizures and convulsions can result.[1]

More than seventy-five years ago, scientists declared magnesium to be an essential mineral. Each year since then, research has revealed more ways in which magnesium is indispensable to life.[2] Yet it is continually being lost from the natural food supply. There has been a gradual decline of dietary magnesium in the United States, from a high of 500 mg/day at the turn of the century to barely 175–225 mg/day today.[3] The

National Academy of Sciences has determined that most Americans are magnesium-deficient, with men obtaining about 80 percent of the recommended daily allowance (RDA) and women averaging only 70 percent.[4] Too few medical researchers and doctors are sounding the alarm, so it is important that you inform yourself and protect your health.[5,6,7]

THE CLINICAL IMPACT OF MAGNESIUM DEFICIENCY

Magnesium was first discovered in huge deposits near a Greek city called Magnesia. Magnesium sulfate, known today as Epsom salts, was used in ancient times as a laxative, and still is to this day. A 1697 medical paper recommended magnesium, with some exaggerated unscientific enthusiasm, for conditions as varied as skin ulcers, depression, vertigo, heartburn, worms, kidney stones, jaundice, and gout. Although we no longer treat all of these conditions specifically with magnesium, current research does support its use for a long list of ailments that you will read about in *The Miracle of Magnesium*.

The amount of research on the topic of magnesium is staggering. To bring you the most current research and medical facts, I've sifted through thousands of pages of scientific studies, each of which begins with the acknowledgment that magnesium is of therapeutic value in treating a myriad of symptoms.

1. *Anxiety and panic attacks.* Magnesium normally helps keep adrenal stress hormones under control.
2. *Asthma.* Both histamine production and bronchial spasms increase with magnesium deficiency.
3. *Blood clots.* Magnesium has an important role to play in preventing blood clots and keeping the blood thin—much like aspirin but without the side effects.
4. *Bowel disease.* Magnesium deficiency slows down the bowel, causing constipation, which could lead to toxicity and malabsorption of nutrients as well as colitis.
5. *Cystitis.* Bladder spasms are worsened by magnesium deficiency.
6. *Depression.* Serotonin, which elevates mood, is dependent on magnesium. A magnesium-deficient brain is also more susceptible to allergens, foreign substances that in rare instances can cause symptoms similar to mental illness.
7. *Detoxification.* Magnesium is crucial for the removal of toxic substances and heavy metals such as aluminum and lead from the body.
8. *Diabetes.* Magnesium enhances insulin secretion, facilitating sugar metabolism. Without magnesium, insulin is not able to transfer glucose into cells. Glucose and insulin build up in the blood, causing various types of tissue damage.
9. *Fatigue.* Magnesium-deficient patients commonly experience fatigue because dozens of enzyme

systems are underfunctioning. An early symptom of magnesium deficiency is fatigue.

10. *Heart disease.* Magnesium deficiency is common in people with heart disease. Magnesium is administered in hospitals for acute myocardial infarction and cardiac arrhythmia. Like any other muscle, the heart requires magnesium. Magnesium is also used to treat angina, or chest pain.

11. *Hypertension.* With insufficient magnesium, blood vessels may go into spasm and cholesterol may rise, both of which lead to blood pressure problems.

12. *Hypoglycemia.* Magnesium keeps insulin under control; without magnesium, episodes of low blood sugar can result.

13. *Insomnia.* Sleep-regulating melatonin production is disturbed without sufficient magnesium.

14. *Kidney disease.* Magnesium deficiency contributes to atherosclerotic kidney failure. Magnesium deficiency creates abnormal lipid levels and worsening blood sugar control in kidney transplant patients.

15. *Migraine.* Serotonin balance is magnesium-dependent. Deficiency of serotonin can result in migraine headaches and depression.

16. *Musculoskeletal conditions.* Fibrositis, fibromyalgia, muscle spasms, eye twitches, cramps, and chronic neck and back pain may be caused by magnesium deficiency and can be relieved with magnesium supplements.

17. *Nerve problems.* Magnesium alleviates peripheral nerve disturbances throughout the body, such as migraines, muscle contractions, gastrointestinal spasms, and calf, foot, and toe cramps. It is also used in treating the central nervous symptoms for vertigo and confusion.

18. *Obstetrical and gynecological problems.* Magnesium helps prevent premenstrual syndrome and dysmenorrhea (cramping pain during menses), is important in the treatment of infertility, and alleviates premature contractions, preeclampsia, and eclampsia in pregnancy. Intravenous magnesium is given in obstetrical wards for pregnancy-induced hypertension and to lessen the risk of cerebral palsy and sudden infant death syndrome (SIDS). Magnesium should be a required supplement for pregnant women.

19. *Osteoporosis.* Use of calcium with vitamin D to enhance calcium absorption without a balancing amount of magnesium causes further magnesium deficiency, which triggers a cascade of events leading to bone loss.

20. *Raynaud's syndrome.* Magnesium helps relax the spastic blood vessels that cause pain and numbness of the fingers.

21. *Tooth decay.* Magnesium deficiency causes an unhealthy balance of phosphorus and calcium in saliva, which damages teeth.

Drugs such as painkillers, diuretics, antibiotics, and cortisone, many of which are inappropriately used for the aforementioned conditions, further deplete magnesium and other minerals, allowing symptoms to get completely out of control. Surgery, malnutrition, third-degree burns, serious injuries, pancreatic inflammation, liver disease, malabsorption disorders, diabetes, hormonal imbalance, and cancer are all seriously stressful medical conditions requiring increased amounts of magnesium.

MY HISTORY WITH MAGNESIUM

In my second year of medical school, I was observing in the obstetrics ward when a young woman in the last stage of labor developed rapidly elevating blood pressure and began convulsing. This was a true medical emergency. Already skeptical about the antihypertensive and anticonvulsant drugs, which had so many side effects and variable results, I wondered what could possibly work that would not be dangerous for the baby. But clearly, this woman needed something both powerful and effective. The attending physician called out for an ampule of magnesium sulfate and immediately injected it into her IV. Within minutes the woman's convulsing had ceased and her blood pressure was returning to normal. I was amazed, and I've never forgotten that miracle of magnesium, which also reinforced my belief that there are safe, effective alternatives to prescription drugs for pain and chronic disease. In addition to my medical school training, I voraciously read all I could find on nutrition and alternative medicine. I even studied acupuncture. Immediately after medical school I embarked upon my naturopathic training. In thirteen years of treating patients, and ten years as a researcher, writer, and consultant, I have frequently found myself acting as an educator, passing on the knowledge of simple, safe treatments and supplements that really work, including magnesium.

But my keen interest in magnesium is personal as well as professional. I had taken a calcium/magnesium supplement for many years, knowing the importance of each to my own health. When I started doing research for this book, however, I realized that my daily heart palpitations, calf muscle cramps at night, and neck and shoulder muscle tension were related to magnesium deficiency. Increasing my dosage from 200 mg a day in a calcium/magnesium combination to 500 mg of magnesium oxide twice a day stopped the palpitations and the cramps and eased the muscle tension considerably.

Magnesium is not some wonder drug touted by a pharmaceutical company in an aggressive marketing campaign. It is a simple element, a mineral vital to life and health, and easily obtained. The more I have learned about magnesium, the more convinced I am that doctors are missing a huge opportunity by not making it one of their "drugs of choice." I hope that by writing this story of magnesium, I will help you keep yourself healthy and at the same time provide an important resource that you can share with your doctor.

PART ONE

The History of Magnesium

CHAPTER 1

The Case for Magnesium:
The Personal History of an Element

Mary joked that she felt as though she was constantly being run over by a slow-moving bus. Cramping in her legs startled her awake at night, making her an insomniac, and she had heart palpitations daily. Her doctor also found that she had high blood sugar—not bad enough to need injections of insulin, but he prescribed pills to try to stimulate more insulin production. Finally, frightening panic attacks came out of nowhere and made this vibrant, fun-loving woman afraid to go outside.

To try to relieve her leg cramps, Mary began taking calcium at night, having read that it was good for cramps and sleep. At first, the calcium seemed to help, but after a week or two, the pains got worse. If she yawned and stretched in bed, her calf muscles would seize up and catapult her to the floor, where she would lie frantically massaging her muscles to try to release the spasm. All the next day, she would limp about with a very tender, bruised feeling in her calf.

Although Mary's heart palpitations had improved some-what after she'd given up her three cups of coffee a day, they too resumed after a few weeks. Every time the palpitations occurred, which was several times a day, they made her cough slightly and catch her breath. She found it frightening, even though her doctor said her stress tests for heart disease were fine and she didn't need further testing with an angiogram.

Both Mary's parents had had adult-onset diabetes, and Mary knew that she should watch her diet, but she was overweight and craved sugary and high-carbohydrate foods that were hard to resist. When the panic attacks hit on top of everything else, Mary knew she had to seek help, and came to my office. She was only fifty-three, far too young to be feeling so bad, and was worried about her future health.

Sam was only forty-nine and experiencing chest pains. At first, he thought they were indigestion, but sometimes the pains would occur in the middle of the night. Concerned, he went to a cardiologist, who found two slightly blocked arteries, not serious enough for bypass surgery. Sam's cholesterol was somewhat elevated, as was his blood pressure, which he attributed to his high-stress occupation and the fact that he had not exercised regularly for the past six months, when he was sidelined with back pain.

The cardiologist observed that his arterial blockage would almost inevitably worsen over time and eventually necessitate surgery. The doctor offered him medication for his high cholesterol, told him not to eat butter or eggs, and gave him nitroglycerine to take whenever he had the pain. If the symptoms got worse, he would prescribe other medications. Sam couldn't imagine having to wait to get worse before doing something about his chest pain; he knew there must be something more he could do to avoid surgery and came to me for advice.

At thirty-five, Jan had actually begun to look forward to going through menopause. That's how bad her PMS symptoms were. As soon as those horrible feelings lifted, she was hit by the sledgehammer of menstrual cramps. She also had migraines, which for years had come before her period but now were occurring once or twice a week. She was so miserable that she was considering a complete hysterectomy, with removal of her hormone-producing ovaries, but wondered whether the migraines, since they were happening all month, were not actually hormonal.

Different as their symptoms are, Mary, Sam, and Jan all suffer from magnesium deficiency. While women and men seem equally susceptible to magnesium deficiency, women may become deficient faster than men due to hormonal fluctuations because pound for pound, they have fewer circulating red blood cells, which carry magnesium, and so perhaps less magnesium available. There are a few other gender differences. Because of magnesium's effect on hormonal regulation and vice versa, women can have deficiencies in pregnancy, when breast-feeding, with premenstrual syndrome (PMS), and with dysmenorrhea (painful periods). Osteoporosis, which affects more women than men, is evidence of a deficiency of both calcium and magnesium. An overactive thyroid, which afflicts more women than men, increases the metabolic rate, which uses up magnesium-requiring ATP (adenosine triphosphate—the energy packets made in each cell in the body). Without magnesium, ATP would not be produced.

Let's follow Mary, Sam, and Jan and see how they overcame their magnesium deficiencies.

When Mary visited me, I charted her health history in detail, according to procedures commonly used by naturopathic doctors, and found several symptoms of magnesium deficiency. In her case it had been made even worse by too much calcium, however, so simple magnesium supplementation wouldn't be enough for Mary. Her diet and lifestyle needed a complete overhaul.

I gave Mary a list of magnesium-rich foods that she needed to start eating, which included nuts, beans, greens, and seeds such as sunflower and pumpkin. Mary realized that she'd been avoiding almost all of these foods: She thought nuts were fattening, beans gave her gas, and greens never seemed fresh enough at the supermarket. She had never even thought about eating seeds.

After a week of enthusiastically eating a lot more magnesium-rich foods, Mary felt somewhat better. To make sure she could get fresh organic greens regularly, she tracked down a local community-supported agriculture (CSA) program and bought a share in a neighboring organic farm. Mary also learned how to soak and cook beans to prevent them from causing gas, and began eating nuts and seeds rich in magnesium and healthy oils, such as almonds, walnuts, pecans, sunflower seeds, and pumpkin seeds.

After her second visit I recommended that she begin taking magnesium supplements. Starting with a dosage of 200 mg a day, we added another 200 mg every two days to build slowly to 600 mg. I cautioned her that it could take months to eliminate magnesium deficiency symptoms and that not all her symptoms would necessarily respond. Within two months, however, Mary was singing the praises of magnesium. Her palpitations and panic attacks had disappeared. Her cravings for sweets were fewer, she was able to control her blood sugar with diet alone, and tests for blood sugar were normal. Her leg cramps were gone, and with them her insomnia. At three months we added calcium along with magnesium so that she would not develop an imbalance of the two. Mary's internist was quite surprised at her improved health and told her to keep up the good work with her diet and supplements.

Sam had an inquiring mind, and I encouraged him to start reading about heart disease. He found that up to

30 percent of angina (chest pain) patients do not have badly blocked arteries but may be suffering from an electrical imbalance that is driven by mineral deficiency, most commonly magnesium.[1] An astonishing 40 to 60 percent of sudden deaths from heart attack may occur in the complete absence of any prior artery blockage, clot formation or heart rhythm abnormalities, most likely from spasms in the arteries (magnesium is a natural antispasmodic).[2,3,4,5] Moreover, he found that magnesium deficiency has been linked to sudden cardiac death. Sam didn't want to wait around for that to happen to him; he was determined to find out what was causing his problem and treat the cause. The more he read, the more intrigued he became. When he read that magnesium deficiency is also associated with muscle pain, especially back pain, that really got his attention, since he had begun having back pain four or five months before he began to develop chest pain.[6]

With a packet of information on magnesium, Sam went back to his cardiologist. Before the doctor saw him, however, a nurse took Sam's blood pressure; it was unusually elevated, even though at home it was usually only a few points above normal. (Doctor-induced hypertension is commonly reported by patients.) The cardiologist swept into the room and immediately began talking about blood pressure medication. Sam countered with magnesium. The cardiologist visibly cooled and said that magnesium was used to control hypertension that occurred in pregnant women because there were no side effects, but that there were plenty of effective drugs for everyone else. When Sam said he would rather not have side effects either, the cardiologist gathered up his file and told him to come back when he was ready to take medications for his heart disease.

When Sam came back to see me, he was still pretty upset by this encounter; he didn't like the specialist refusing to discuss a possible magnesium deficiency as part of the picture. Sam and I agreed that magnesium seemed the best treatment for him to initiate at this time since he was not willing to take medications.

Sam began adding magnesium to his diet by eating magnesium-rich foods. After a week he felt much calmer, but he still had chest and back pain. So he added magnesium and calcium supplements, and in about three months he felt almost normal.

Among the studies Sam read was one that looked at the correspondence between type A personalities and magnesium deficiency. From the description, Sam realized he was a type A, an aggressive guy who lived on adrenaline, time pressure, and stress. This type of behavior drains the body of magnesium and can lead to disorders such as heart disease, muscle spasms, hypersensitivity, and irritability.[7] Prolonged psychological stress raises adrenaline, the stress hormone, which depletes magnesium.[8] Both Sam's back and chest pain would hit when he was under stress. So Sam worked on ways to control his stress and added more magnesium when he knew he couldn't avoid it. On days when he exercised, Sam added an extra 200 mg of magnesium to his diet, since sweat loss during heavy exercise (cycling and jogging) and working in the heat deplete magnesium. Just drinking water won't replace all the minerals lost. By paying attention to the many factors that affected his mind-body health, Sam lowered his cholesterol and stress levels and reduced his chance of a heart attack and of needing surgery to unblock his arteries.

Jan heard that yoga might help her PMS and painful periods, and she really needed to learn to relax, so she took classes at a local health club. The teacher also ran regular detox and cooking classes, which Jan decided to join when she realized she didn't have to "give up everything" and become a vegetarian. One of the first things Jan learned in the detox class was the importance of having regular bowel movements. Jan was lucky if she had one a week. If the bowel doesn't empty once a day, toxins can be reabsorbed back into the body from the colon. The longer debris sits in the colon, the more fluid is reabsorbed, making stools solid and difficult to pass. PMS and endometriosis, which causes painful periods, are considered by some natural-health experts to worsen with constipation and toxicity.[9]

During cooking classes, Jan faced the fact that she was a junk food addict. Magnesium is necessary in hundreds of enzymes in the body but is almost totally lost during the processing of packaged and fast foods. The older women in her class were suffering from a variety of problems that included cancer, heart disease, and osteoporosis. Is that how she would end up in ten or twenty years if she didn't take care of her health now? Learning how many basic nutrients she lacked in her diet made her marvel that she wasn't even more ill. Her new diet included greens, beans, nuts, and seeds, which cleared up her constipation and almost eliminated her PMS and painful periods. When she came to see me on the advice of her yoga teacher, it was clear she was on the right track. I recommended that she begin taking a magnesium supplement along with calcium and a multiple vitamin; with all her lifestyle changes, she felt like a new person.

MAGNESIUM, THE SPARK OF LIFE

In a poetic reference to magnesium's crucial role in evolution, Dr. Jerry Aikawa of the University of Colorado calls magnesium the ur-mineral, the most important mineral to man and all living organisms.[10] It is critical to the metabolic processes of lowly one-celled living organisms and is the second most abundant element inside human cells. Magnesium existed at the beginning of life and was involved with all aspects of cell production and growth. When plants evolved to use the sun as their energy source, magnesium played a pivotal role in the development of chlorophyll. So in both plants and animals, magnesium became an essential mineral involved in hundreds of enzyme processes affecting every aspect of life.

Presently, seventeen minerals are considered essential

for human life, and it is quite possible that more minerals will be found to be indispensable as we take more time to study life's mineral connection. Ninety-nine percent of the body's mineral content is made up of seven macrominerals: sodium, potassium, calcium, phosphorus, chlorine, sulfur, and magnesium. The other 1 percent comprises ten trace minerals. As with most minerals, the element magnesium occurs in nature combined with other elements. It joins naturally with sulfur to make Epsom salts (magnesium sulfate), with carbon to make magnesium carbonate, and with calcium to make dolomite. Magnesium is also found in partnership with silica in talc and asbestos. Like calcium, it is an alkaline mineral, which neutralizes acid, and some magnesium compounds are antacids used to treat heartburn.

My first encounter with magnesium was in high school chemistry. Each student was given a thin strip of magnesium and told to light one end carefully. The previous week we had learned that magnesium is the eighth most abundant element, constituting approximately 2 percent of the earth's crust and 1.14 percent of seawater. By comparison, calcium makes up 3 percent of the earth's crust but only 0.05 percent of seawater. There are 4–6 tsp (20–28 g or 2 oz) of magnesium in the body, comprising about 0.05 percent of the body's weight. This information in no way prepared us for the dynamic effect of lighting the magnesium strip. It flared up like an electric sparkler and disappeared in a flash. This effervescent property serves as an important reminder of magnesium's versatility as the spark of life, constantly igniting metabolic reactions throughout the body.

THE BODY IS ELECTRIC

The impulses for any and all movement in the body arise from electrical transmission. These microcurrents of electricity that pass along the nerves were first measured in 1966. Scientists soon discovered that the conductor for these bodily electrical currents was calcium and that magnesium was necessary to maintain the proper level of calcium in the blood.[11] More recent research indicates that calcium enters the cells by way of calcium channels that are jealously guarded by magnesium. Magnesium allows a certain amount of calcium to enter a cell to create the necessary electrical transmission, and then immediately helps to eject the calcium once the work is done. Why? If calcium accumulates in the cell, it causes toxicity and disrupts cell function. Too much calcium entering cells can cause symptoms of heart disease (such as angina, high blood pressure, and arrhythmia), asthma, or headaches. Magnesium is nature's calcium channel blocker.[12,13,14]

About 60–65 percent of all our magnesium is housed in our bones and teeth. The remaining 35–40 percent is found in the rest of the body, including muscle and tissue cells and body fluids. The highest concentrations are in the heart and brain cells, so it is no wonder that the major symptoms of magnesium deficiency affect the heart and brain. These are also the two organs that have considerable electrical activity measured by EKG (electrocardiogram) and EEG (electroencephalogram). Our blood contains only *1 percent* of the body's total magnesium.

Magnesium mostly works inside our tissue cells, producing ATP energy packets for our body's vital force and triggering production of all the body's protein structures by revving up messenger RNA. It is also a requirement for the production of DNA, our genetic code. Both of the basic building blocks of life, RNA and DNA, are dependent on magnesium to maintain stable genes.[15] In addition to its stabilizing effect on DNA and the structure of chromosomes, magnesium is an essential cofactor in almost all enzyme systems involved in the processing of DNA. Research shows that without sufficient magnesium, DNA synthesis becomes sluggish.

WHAT DOES MAGNESIUM DO?

Magnesium's hundreds of activities in the human body can be divided into five essential categories:[16]

1. Magnesium is a cofactor assisting enzymes in catalyzing most chemical reactions in the body, including temperature regulation.
2. Magnesium produces and transports energy.
3. Magnesium is necessary for the synthesis of protein.

4. Magnesium helps to transmit nerve signals.
5. Magnesium helps to relax muscles.

1. COFACTOR IN CHEMICAL REACTIONS

Enzymes are protein molecules that stimulate every chemical reaction in the body. Magnesium is required to make hundreds of these enzymes work.

2. PRODUCING AND TRANSPORTING ENERGY

Magnesium and the B-complex vitamins are excellent examples of energy nutrients, because they activate enzymes that control digestion, absorption, and the utilization of proteins, fats, and carbohydrates. Because magnesium is involved with hundreds of enzymatic reactions throughout the body, deficiency can affect every aspect of life and cause a score of symptoms. Of the 325 magnesium-dependent enzymes, the most important enzyme reaction involves the creation of energy by activating adenosine triphosphate (ATP), the fundamental energy storage molecule of the body. ATP may be what the Chinese refer to as *qi* or life force. Magnesium is required for the body to produce and store energy. Without magnesium there is no energy, no movement, no life. It is that simple.

3. SYNTHESIZING PROTEIN

Magnesium is used in synergy with dozens of other vitamins and minerals to create structural components of the body. Under the direction of magnesium, enzymes and nutrients modify the building blocks from food to create the body. Without magnesium, there is no body. RNA and DNA, which contain the genetic blueprints for the formation of all the protein molecules in the body, are also dependent on magnesium.

4. TRANSMITTING NERVE SIGNALS

Magnesium permits calcium to enter a nerve cell to allow electrical transmission along the nerves to and from the brain. Even our thoughts, via brain neurons, are dependent on magnesium.

5. RELAXING MUSCLES

Calcium causes contraction in skeletal muscle fibers, and magnesium causes relaxation. When there is too much calcium and insufficient magnesium, you can get sustained muscle contraction: twitches, spasms, and even convulsions. Smooth muscles directed by too much calcium and insufficient magnesium can tighten the bronchial tract, causing asthma; cause cramping in the uterus and painful periods; and cause spasms in blood vessels, resulting in hypertension.

THE DANCE OF CALCIUM AND MAGNESIUM

Calcium and magnesium share equal importance in our bodies. Newton's law says that for every action there is an equal and opposite reaction, and calcium and magnesium dance within this law. Neither can act without eliciting a reaction from the other. At the biochemical level, magnesium and calcium are known to act antagonistically towards each other. Many enzymes whose activities critically depend on a sufficient amount of intracellular magnesium will be detrimentally affected by small increases in levels of cellular calcium. Growth of cells, cell division, and intermediary metabolism are also absolutely dependent on the availability of magnesium, which can be compromised if excess calcium is present.[17]

To understand how you can create a calcium/magnesium imbalance in your own body, try this experiment in your kitchen. Crush a calcium pill and see how much dissolves in 1 oz of water. Then crush a magnesium pill and slowly stir it into the calcium water. When you introduce the magnesium, the remaining calcium dissolves; it becomes more water-soluble. The same thing happens in your bloodstream, heart, brain, kidneys, and all the tissues in your body. If you don't have enough magnesium to help keep calcium dissolved, you may end up with calcium-excess muscle spasms, fibromyalgia, hardening of the arteries, and even dental cavities. Another scenario plays out in the kidneys. If there is too much calcium in the kidneys and not enough magnesium to dissolve it, you can get kidney stones.

All muscles, including the heart and blood vessels, contain more magnesium than calcium. If magnesium is deficient, calcium floods the smooth muscle cells of the blood vessels and causes spasms leading to constricted blood vessels and therefore higher blood pressure, arterial spasm, angina, and heart attack.[18] A proper balance of magnesium in relation to calcium can prevent these symptoms. Calcium excess, stimulating the cells in the muscular layer of the temporal arteries over the temples, can cause migraine headaches. Excess calcium can constrict the smooth muscle surrounding the small airways of the lung, causing restricted breathing and asthma. Finally, too much calcium, without the protective effect of magnesium, can irritate delicate nerve cells of the brain. Cells that are irritated by calcium fire electrical impulses repeatedly, depleting their energy stores and causing cell death.

THE CALCIUM DISTRACTION

The irony of the calcium-magnesium story is that without magnesium calcium will not work properly. Both our current diet and tendency to oversupplement with calcium, however, make getting enough magnesium almost impossible. Research shows that the ratio of calcium to magnesium in the paleolithic or caveman diet—the ancient diet that had evolved with our bodies—was 1:1, compared with a 5:1 to 15:1 ratio in present-day diets.[19] With an average of ten times more calcium than magnesium in our current diet, there is no doubt about widespread magnesium deficiency in modern times.

The emphasis on calcium supplementation has diverted our attention from any other mineral, even though all minerals are crucial to the proper functioning of the body.

In our society we tend to look for "the best," "the most important," "the star," and forget that it takes a team and teamwork to get anything accomplished, including body processes. Calcium, because it is the most abundant mineral in the body, therefore became "the star." Even though research has accumulated on magnesium over the past four decades, it has never been adequately publicized and discussed.

CHAPTER 2

Magnesium: The Missing Mineral

A 1988 U.S. government study concluded that the standard American diet failed to provide the daily requirement of magnesium.[1] That was a decade and a half ago, and you can be sure that most people get even less today, when junk food makes up 27 percent of our diet. Mildred Seelig, M.D., and many other magnesium experts have also come to the inescapable conclusion that the typical American diet, which is rich in fat, sugar, salt, synthetic vitamin D, phosphates, protein, fiber, and supplemented calcium, actually *increases* the need for dietary magnesium. In 1997, the National Academy of Sciences found that *most* Americans are magnesium-deficient. When men obtain only 80 percent of the minimum requirement of magnesium to run innumerable body functions and women at 70 percent get even less of what they absolutely need, then our bodies are just not able to function properly.[2]

Let's look at some of the reasons you may be lacking in magnesium.

PROCESSED FOOD LACKS MAGNESIUM

During the refining and processing of food, significant amounts of magnesium can be lost. The process of extracting oils from magnesium-rich nuts and seeds strips away this essential mineral. Nearly all the magnesium in grains is lost during the milling process to make flour. Chemicals that are used in the preparation of frozen vegetables to preserve their rich green color result in a lowered magnesium content. Finally, in the kitchen, when vegetables are boiled, magnesium leaches out into the water.

PERCENTAGE OF MAGNESIUM LOST DURING FOOD PROCESSING

Refining of flour from wheat	80 percent
Polishing of rice	83 percent
Production of starch from corn	97 percent
Extraction of white sugar from molasses	99 percent

What can we do to defend our magnesium sources? It is best to buy organic foods, eat as many raw vegetables as possible, and when you do cook vegetables, quickly steam them for only a few minutes until they are slightly cooked but still crisp. You can also save the nutrient-filled water to use as soup stock.

STOMACH ACID IS ESSENTIAL FOR MAGNESIUM ABSORPTION

Inefficient stomach digestion and intestinal absorption can lead to deficiencies of magnesium. When you are under serious physical or even emotional stress, your body might not produce sufficient stomach acid, which is required for digestion and for chemically changing minerals into an absorbable form. The elderly as well as people with arthritis, asthma, depression, diabetes, gallbladder disease, osteoporosis, or gum disease are often deficient in hydrochloric acid.[3] All these conditions are also associated with magnesium deficiency.

On the other hand, America's number one over-the-counter drug type is antacids. Heartburn and indigestion, the result of bad eating habits, plague the nation. But the "cure" in this case is no better than the disease. The roiling and burning in the gut from sugary junk food and greasy fast food is being inappropriately blamed on too much stomach acid. In many cases, heartburn is due to fermentation in the stomach and a backflow of pancreatic enzymes from the small intestine.[4] By neutralizing normal stomach acids, antacids make it impossible for us to absorb minerals or digest our food properly. Our magnesium can be even further depleted if we use calcium carbonate antacids because the calcium they contain causes more magnesium to be excreted.

ABSORPTION OF DIETARY MAGNESIUM HINDERED

Magnesium is ultimately absorbed into the bloodstream from the small intestine. In general, an average of only 50 percent of ingested magnesium is absorbed; the rest is eliminated in the stool or urine. A number of conditions influence the degree of absorption:

- Whether the intestines are healthy or diseased
- Availability of the protein transport molecule for magnesium
- Availability of parathyroid hormone
- The rate of water absorption, because magnesium is soluble in water
- The amounts of calcium, phosphorus, potassium, sodium, and lactose (milk sugar) in the body, all of which inhibit magnesium absorption
- Supplemental iron, which can impede magnesium absorption and vice versa (if you take both, you should take them several hours apart)

MAGNESIUM BLOCKED BY CERTAIN FOODS

A food may be high or low in magnesium, but you should also know that certain foods contain magnesium antagonists, such as oxalic acid, which is found in spinach and chard, or phytic acid, found in the hulls and bran of seeds and grains. Oxalic acid and phytic acid can form insoluble compounds with magnesium, causing it to be eliminated rather than absorbed. Saturated fats (from meat and cheese) can bind with mineral compounds in food, making insoluble clumps of fat that end up forming plaque in your arteries and blood vessels (atherosclerosis) and can eventually raise your blood pressure and lead to heart disease. Taking magnesium supplements with a fatty meal is a waste. Magnesium supplements are best taken on an empty stomach.

There is much evidence that a high-protein diet only makes magnesium deficiency worse, and if you are following such a regimen, you should take at least 300 mg of supplemental magnesium.[5]

Soybeans, too, are high in phytic acid, which intercepts minerals from all foods and blocks their uptake and absorption in the intestinal tract. People who depend on grains and legumes as their main source of protein often have mineral deficiencies. Soy has one of the highest phytate levels of any legume and, unlike others, its phytic acid is not destroyed with extended cooking time. Only fermentation (as is done in the production of miso and *tempeh*) will reduce the phytic acid levels of soy.

Vegetarians, who substitute unfermented tofu for meat and dairy, risk having severe mineral deficiencies. Moreover, the menopausal population may be overusing soy (for its natural phytoestrogenic effects) and developing similar mineral deficiencies. As a cheap alternative to meat, soy (as soy protein isolate and textured vegetable protein) has exploded on the school lunch scene and in the fast-food industry. Too much soy can cause mineral deficiencies in children, who really need their minerals to build strong bones and teeth—the structure for adult health.

A JUNK-FOOD DIET IS NOT
A MAGNESIUM DIET

Even in a healthy diet with proper protein intake, the addition of 150 mg of elemental magnesium a day can make dramatic changes in health.[6] (See Chapter 13 for a full discussion of magnesium supplementations.) If a good diet can leave you magnesium-deficient, a poor diet can seriously undermine your health.

We live in strange times, when people avidly watch gourmet-cooking shows while devouring junk food. Junk food provides 27 percent of most people's daily calories; an astounding 90 percent of our food dollar is spent on processed foods. People who eat primarily in institutions, such as hospitals, colleges, or hotels, tend to consume only cooked and processed foods and are likely to be magnesium-deficient, as are people who drink only soft water because water-softening agents eliminate magnesium.[7] Fluoridated water is deficient in magnesium, and distilled water pulls minerals out of the tissues and flushes them out of the body. People who drink soda and soft drinks may also be magnesium-deficient because sugar uses up magnesium.[8,9] Carbonated beverages and processed foods (luncheon meats and hot dogs) contain phosphates, which bind with magnesium to make insoluble magnesium phosphate, which is not absorbed by the body. People who consume more than three alcoholic drinks a day can also be deficient because alcohol blocks absorption and enhances excretion of magnesium.[10] Coffee also acts as a diuretic, which hastens magnesium out of the body. Dieting to lose weight, especially by using diuretics, can drain the body of magnesium and is very unhealthy.

MAGNESIUM-DEFICIENT SOIL RESULTS IN DEFICIENCY

Even if you try to eat magnesium-rich foods, you can still come up short because the soil itself is deficient in magnesium. Magnesium is found in vegetables, nuts, seeds, and whole grains, but this is true only under optimal growing conditions. Plants grown on depleted soil on factory farms contain very little magnesium because it is not routinely included in fertilizer. If there is no magnesium in the soil, plants will have none; they cannot manufacture it out of thin air. So don't believe it when someone says that you can get all your nutrients in a good, balanced diet. That may be true only if you eat organic food and only if the organic farmers use a full spectrum of nutrients in their fertilizer, including magnesium. To get enough magnesium in your diet today, you probably need to take supplements.

DRUGS CAUSE MAGNESIUM DEFICIENCY

Ironically, one of the foremost magnesium experts, Mildred Seelig, M.D., began her research career over forty years ago working for drug companies. It was there she first noticed that many of the side effects of drugs were actually magnesium deficiency symptoms. It seemed to her that many drugs cause increased demand for and utilization of magnesium— for example, by creating acidity in the body, which then draws on available magnesium from the cells to try to neutralize the acid and minimize its toxic effects. Other drugs seemed to deplete magnesium from the body or, conversely, manifest their positive effects because they increase the level of magnesium in the body.[11]

The following drugs can create magnesium deficiencies:[12]

- Common diuretics
- Birth control pills
- Insulin
- Digitalis, prescribed for some heart conditions
- Tetracycline and certain other antibiotics
- Cortisone

DRUG INTERACTIONS WITH MAGNESIUM

Other drugs interact with magnesium in specific ways.[13] For example, magnesium is a muscle relaxant, so it enhances the actions of prescription muscle relaxants such as tubocurarine (used in surgery), barbiturates, hypnotics, and narcotics. These medications may be decreased under a doctor's supervision if you are on magnesium. Tell your anesthesiologist before surgery if you are taking magnesium supplements.

Magnesium protects the kidneys, so it may be beneficial during treatment with aminoglycoside antibiotics (which result in magnesium wasting) and immunosuppressant drugs such as cyclosporin and cisplatin. Discuss this with your doctor.

Diuretics and cardiac drugs waste magnesium. Additional magnesium intake is recommended during administration of diuretics and cardiac glycosides. Check with your doctor.

Magnesium inhibits the absorption of iron, tetracyclines, ciprofloxacin, vancomycin, isoniazid, chlorpromazine, trimethoprim, nitrofurantoin, and sodium fluoride. Take these medications two to three hours before or after magnesium supplements. (Sodium fluoride is prescribed for osteoporosis—although taking magnesium may be a wiser choice; see Chapter 8.)

WHY HAVEN'T WE HEARD
ABOUT MAGNESIUM?

The vast majority of us were not exposed to nutritional education in school. But what about doctors? As you may suspect, doctors generally do not learn about nutrition or nutrient supplementation in medical school because they are studying disease, not wellness. When you visit a medical doctor, you may think you are going there to improve your health or prevent illness, but doctors have little time to educate their patients about how to keep themselves well. And patients often will not change their lifestyle unless their doctor tells them to, believing that if vitamins were so important, the doctor would have told them to take supplements. (Of course, some patients don't change the way they live even when their doctor does tell them they have to lose weight and eat right.)

WHEN ALL YOU HAVE IS A HAMMER

In the first two years of medical school I learned all about diseases; the second two years I studied drug treatments for those diseases. We spent no time on nutrient deficiencies. Have you heard the expression "When all you have is a hammer, everything begins to look like a nail"? That is very much the case with doctors and drug treatments. But even worse, with thousands of drugs in the pharmaceutical compendium, it is quite impossible for doctors to keep up on the latest drugs, and impossible to prevent side effects or serious drug interactions. And although allopathic medicine is said to be scientific, most patients are on more than one drug at a time, and there are *no* studies proving the safety of drug combinations.

According to magnesium expert Mildred Seelig, M.D., while a tremendous amount of magnesium research has been done in India, Britain, France, and other European countries, doctors in the United States use the excuse that not enough research has been done here for them to feel informed enough to prescribe it. Dr. Seelig calls this the "not-invented-here syndrome." Pioneers such as Drs. Bella and Burton Altura, however, continue to do original magnesium research in this country. Every year for the past forty years they have produced on average a dozen peer-reviewed journal articles on magnesium and ionic magnesium testing. Their research convinces even die-hard skeptics—when they take the time to become informed—of the clear need for magnesium supplementation and the absolute requirement for accurate testing.

DRUG COMPANIES FUND DRUG RESEARCH, NOT MINERAL RESEARCH

Medical science studies one symptom at a time, in isolation, and generally tries to find one cause for that symptom and one drug that treats it. The bias of medical research makes it search for a drug that will eventually pay for the costly studies necessary to bring it to market. Everyone agrees that magnesium is indispensable for health, disease prevention, and all life processes, but it has been ignored because there is no money in selling a common nutrient. Magnesium cannot be patented, so pharmaceutical companies do not engage in magnesium research. There is no advertising budget for magnesium, compared to the hundreds of millions of dollars spent on advertising prescription drugs; nutrients do not get media attention. To make matters worse, over the past two decades the bulk of university funding has come from the pharmaceutical industry, which primarily funds drug research.[14] Scientific medicine ignores nutrient investigation in favor of drugs. Older research is also ignored by health providers. Doctors may have heard years ago that magnesium offered some promise in heart disease, but they haven't read any new studies, so they assume that the treatment must have not panned out.

Doctors seem to be waiting for a large clinical trial, for example, following twenty thousand people taking magnesium for life. It would have been nice if such a study had been initiated thirty years ago. I would suggest starting one now, but I don't know who would pay for such a trial. And do we have the luxury of waiting for those results? No. Do we presently know enough about magnesium to recommend widespread supplementation? Yes.

An analysis of seven major clinical studies shows that intravenous magnesium reduced the risk of death by 55 percent after acute heart attack. These results were published in the prestigious *British Medical Journal* and the widely read *Drugs*.[15,16] As I've noted, Drs. Bella and Burton Altura have been researching magnesium and its clinical application for over forty years.[17] The ionized magnesium electrode, produced by Nova Biomedical (Waltham, MA) at the Alturas' urging and tested at State University of New York has given doctors a reliable magnesium test and taken the guesswork out of diagnosing magnesium deficiency.[18] Dr. Alexander Mauskaup, working with the Alturas, has proven the connection between migraines and magnesium many times over and puts magnesium treatment into practice at the New York Headache Center.[19,20,21] Dr. Mildred Seelig has contributed comprehensive reviews of magnesium at New York Medical College, the American College of Nutrition, and more recently at the Department of Nutrition, University of North Carolina.[22,23] Dr. Jean Durlach, president of the International Society for the Development of Research on Magnesium (SDRM), editor in chief of *Magnesium Research*, and professor at St. Vincent de Paul Hospital in Paris, has done extensive reviews of ongoing magnesium research.[24,25] Magnesium researchers agree that we no longer need to sit on the sidelines or reserve judgment on the benefits of magnesium; we need to implement what we know, *now*.

PART TWO

Magnesium-Deficient Conditions

CHAPTER 3

Anxiety, Pain, and Magnesium
for Athletes

THREE THINGS YOU NEED TO KNOW ABOUT
MAGNESIUM, ANXIETY, AND DEPRESSION

1. Magnesium deficiency can produce symptoms of anxiety or depression, including muscle weakness, fatigue, eye twitches, insomnia, anorexia, apathy, apprehension, poor memory, confusion, anger, nervousness, and rapid pulse.
2. Serotonin, the "feel-good" brain chemical that is boosted by Prozac, depends on magnesium for its production and function.
3. Magnesium supports our adrenal glands, which are overworked by stress.

Each year millions of people are introduced to the merry-go-round of psychiatric drugs and psychological counseling for symptoms that may in fact be rooted in magnesium deficiency. Additional millions try unsuccessfully to cope with their problems by turning to alcohol, street drugs, and other addictive behavior to suppress their pain. We are a nation suffering a 32 percent incidence of anxiety, depression, and drug problems. Social epidemiologist Myrna Weissman at Columbia University reports that more and more Americans are becoming depressed, getting depressed at a younger age, and experiencing more severe and frequent periods of depression. Each generation born in the twentieth century has suffered more depression than the previous one, and since World War II the overall rate of depression has more than doubled.[1,2] A recent study in the *Archives of General Psychiatry* showed a doubling of depression in women from 1970 to 1992, with the use of psychiatric drugs skyrocketing as a result. Children are not immune: American schoolchildren today are taking four times as many psychiatric medications as in all of the rest of the world combined.[3]

People do not get anxiety, panic attacks, or depression because they have a deficiency of Valium or Prozac. Our bodies do not require these substances for essential metabolic processes. However, we can develop a myriad of psychological symptoms because of a deficiency of magnesium, something our bodies do require. Does it make any sense to merely switch our addictions from sugar, alcohol, drugs, and cigarettes to prescription medication without looking at the possible underlying metabolic causes? Psychiatrists all too often rely on prescription drugs for suffering patients and have no insight into the metabolic functions of the mind and body and what happens when nutrients are deficient. Anxiety and depression are often nutrient deficiency diseases and chemical sensitivities, *not* drug deficiency diseases.

Darcy had driven across a mile-long bridge every day for years, so why one morning did she suddenly feel as though she would die if she didn't pull over? She was sweating and her heart was pounding; she felt sick to her stomach and couldn't get her breath. What was happening to her? Fortunately, she had her cell phone and called her best friend, Sara, who helped her calm herself and breathe her way across the bridge safely. Later, while talking with Sara to try to make sense of the episode, Darcy said she had been on a liquid protein diet for a few weeks. Sara pointed out that it could have thrown something out of balance, and she reminded Darcy that she had warned her of the dangers of this type of diet.

The two women reviewed the list of supplements that Darcy had been taking as part of the program and found that she had neglected to take the magnesium that had been suggested. Sara grabbed a natural health encyclopedia and, sure enough, magnesium deficiency was listed as one of the possible causes of panic attacks.

If Sara had read further, she would have found that the body demands more magnesium when on a liquid protein diet and that the dangers of such a diet have been documented for decades.[4] By eating only protein, which has little magnesium, Darcy had set herself up for a terrifying attack. Fortunately, she discovered this before pursuing a prescription for a tranquilizer to deal with the frightening symptoms of panic attack.

Lack of magnesium may not have been the only cause of Darcy's panic attack. Her high-protein diet could easily have led to hypoglycemia. When blood sugar (glucose) is low, the body reacts with a surge of adrenaline to bring glucose levels back to normal, in order to keep this essential nutrient fueling the brain. Adrenaline acts to speed the heart and retrieve glucose from liver storage. Sometimes people perceive a normal adrenaline rush as a panic attack. Interestingly enough, magnesium is also required for blood sugar control.

Women tend to pay attention to their feelings and interpret symptoms such as panic attacks as signs of emotional imbalance, for which they seek support. The support they get, however, is often in the form of a prescription for an antianxiety drug instead of sound advice to eat a better diet, exercise, and take the right balance of supplements.

Magnesium deficiency can be an underlying cause of anxiety and depression, as determined in several clinical trials.[5] Symptoms of chronic magnesium deficiency include anxious behavior, hyperemotionality, apathy, apprehension, poor memory, confusion, anger, nervousness, muscle weakness, fatigue, headaches, insomnia, light-headedness, dizziness, nervous fits, the feeling of a lump in the throat, impaired breathing, muscle cramps (including leg cramps), a tingling or pricking or creeping feeling on the skin, rapid pulse, chest pain, palpitations, and abnormal heart rhythm.[6,7]

ANXIETY

Stress is so prevalent in our daily life that we have become desensitized to it and the message it is trying to give us, which is to slow down. Anxiety is a chemical reaction created when the adrenal glands respond to a stressful event, such as low blood sugar, by releasing adrenaline. Adrenaline is very useful if you're trying to escape from a dangerous situation, because it gives you that fight-or-flight response: the heart starts pumping faster; digestion slows down; energy stores are released from the liver and made available to the heart, lungs, and muscles; and the muscles of the arms and legs are activated. All of these responses require magnesium. So each time we experience any kind of stress, our magnesium stores are tapped to create energy. This magnesium depletion itself stresses the body, which can result in panic attacks, which equals yet more stress. Not only do our overworked adrenals cause magnesium depletion, but even more adrenaline is released under stress when magnesium levels are low in the body, leaving people feeling irritable, nervous, edgy, or even ready to explode. It's the proverbial catch-22.[8] To put an end to anxiety, magnesium needs to be replaced.

During stress reactions, calcium is also required to stimulate the release of adrenaline. A calcium excess, however, causes a *flood* of adrenaline. Sufficient magnesium will buffer excess calcium and keep it within normal levels, limiting the stress response. Magnesium is important because it naturally diminishes the excitability of the nervous system and lowers the level of calcium around nerve cells. This function of magnesium is also significant in heart disease and other stress-induced illness.[9,10]

CHRONIC STRESS

According to Hans Selye, the Canadian doctor famous for his work on stress in the 1960s, magnesium is also depleted when the body shifts from a short-term fight-or-flight reaction to a chronic stress reaction. The adrenal glands produce cortisol, a type of cortisone, and another stress hormone, norepinephrine, that acts like adrenaline and also causes magnesium depletion.

Chronic stress can come from feeling insecure and threatened, or from exposure to toxic chemicals, heavy metals, or even loud noise, which assaults the nervous system and overworks the immune system. For example, constant loud noise in an industrial work setting induced a significant increase of total serum magnesium (as magnesium was released from tissues) and significantly increased urinary excretion of magnesium, indicating a magnesium deficiency, which lasted for forty-eight hours after exposure.[11]

MAGNESIUM-DEFICIENT KIDS

It's not just adults who can get anxious because of magnesium-deficient diets. Our children are also susceptible when their favorite foods are magnesium-deficient hot dogs, pizza, and soda. The stress in their lives—from peer pressure, academic and athletic performance pressures, worries about body image, the changes and hormonal fluctuations of puberty, exposure to negative events and violence through the media—also contributes. Children are underdiagnosed when it comes to magnesium deficiency, but can have magnesium deficiencies for the same reasons as adults. Attention deficit hyperactivity disorder (ADHD), juvenile delinquency, and childhood depression are associated with magnesium deficiency, and some say these conditions can be caused by it.[12] Instead of reaching for Ritalin or Prozac for kids, consider whether they're getting enough magnesium first.

Dr. Leo Galland, author of *Superimmunity for Kids*, speculates that hyperactive children need extra magnesium due to their constantly high adrenaline levels. Dr. Galland recommends 6 mg per pound of weight per day (for example, 240 mg for a 40-pound child). Because magnesium is hard to find in a form suitable for young children, he suggests 1 tbsp of magnesium citrate a day or 1½ tsp of milk of magnesia a day. These are both laxatives in much larger doses, but in such small doses they supply the necessary magnesium without a laxative effect.[13]

SEROTONIN, MAGNESIUM, AND DEPRESSION

You may be familiar with serotonin, the body's natural "feel-good" brain chemical. Magnesium is important in the serotonin story because it is a necessary contributor for release and the uptake of serotonin by brain cells. With proper amounts of magnesium, nature makes sufficient serotonin and you experience emotional balance. But when stress depletes magnesium, a vicious cycle spins out of control, and depression can occur. The body needs magnesium in order to release and bind adequate amounts of serotonin in the brain.

The pharmaceutical industry has focused its research for the treatment of depression on selective serotonin reuptake inhibitors (SSRIs) such as Prozac to capitalize on serotonin's chemical effects instead of giving serotonin what it really needs—magnesium. SSRIs create artificially elevated levels of serotonin in the body by preventing its breakdown and elimination; serotonin lingers longer in the brain and theoretically causes mood elevation. This is what is *supposed* to happen, but everyone has a different reaction to the manipulation of their brain chemicals. For some people, prolonged, rising levels of serotonin can liberate them from a long depression. For others, the drug can lead to anxiety and irritability. Another group of people tend to have flattened moods in which they can neither weep nor laugh, keeping them from the extremes of depression or mania but relegating them to a one-dimensional life.

This was Maggie's situation. She was on Prozac and desperately trying to come off it because she was unable to cry or experience real emotions. Maggie was down to one-quarter of a tablet but was afraid to stop in case her depression came back. She also had high blood pressure, high cholesterol, periodic muscle cramps, and constipation. I asked her to have her magnesium tested, and her cardiologist said it was normal; he said she didn't need magnesium but should continue to take her five prescription medications to control her symptoms. She called me when her G.P. thought her muscle cramps were a major blood clot in the leg. We didn't have time to ship a blood sample to the lab that performs ionized magnesium testing, so I encouraged her to take 300 mg of magnesium twice a day and go for a Doppler scan to rule out blood clots. Fortunately, the scan was negative, so Maggie was able to avoid several more medications to treat blood clots, and the magnesium was already working to relieve her symptoms. Within two weeks Maggie was also off the Prozac and able to cry again.

TREATMENT FOR ANXIETY AND DEPRESSION

DIET

Avoid food additives, artificial sweeteners, sugar, and wheat. Eat a whole-foods diet—organic, if possible—and avoid processed and junk food.

SUPPLEMENTS

Magnesium: 300 mg twice a day

Calcium: 800–1,000 mg daily

B complex: 5–50 mg per day (derived in whole or in part from natural sources such as brewer's yeast, wheat germ, or liver)

5-hydroxytryptamine: 50–100 mg half an hour before meals, three times a day (this is an amino acid that crosses the blood-brain barrier and is naturally converted into serotonin; it has the same action as Prozac but no side effects)

St. John's wort: 300 mg of standardized extract three times a day

SLEEP AIDS

Melatonin: 2–3 mg one hour before bedtime

5-hydroxytryptamine: 50–200 mg, one half hour before bedtime, on an empty stomach

Hops, valerian, and skullcap herbal combinations: one or two 500 mg capsules before bedtime

STRESS RELEASE

Exercise is excellent for both anxiety and depression (try yoga, walking, biking, Pilates, swimming), as are meditation, long baths, journal writing, and Emotional Freedom Techniques (EFT, information available at www. emofree.com).

Because depression can be so debilitating, even life-threatening, I understand why doctors feel it requires strong measures to combat it, but these strong measures don't always work. The alternative that many doctors are missing is the nutrient connection. Magnesium deficiency is a potential cause for every type of depression. All treatment protocols should begin with adequate doses of this valuable mineral.[14]

RAYNAUD'S SYNDROME

Sally had terrible leg cramps. During the night, her legs felt jumpy and twitchy and kept her awake. If she did fall asleep, muscle cramps in her calf would wake her up. In addition her fingers began turning white, blue, and red. A young internist diagnosed her as having Raynaud's syndrome, a circulatory condition caused by the spasm of tiny arteries, especially in the hands and feet.

Raynaud's syndrome may occur suddenly or as a result

of other chronic illnesses such as connective tissue disease, trauma, or pulmonary hypertension, in which cases it is called Raynaud's phenomenon. Raynaud's syndrome is seen mostly in young women and rarely leads to damage of the extremities. Cold is often the only stimulus that initiates the blood vessel spasms, which may last from minutes to hours. Emotional stress can also play a role in bringing on an attack. Besides the noted color changes there can be agonizing pain, especially when the fingers are rewarming. Symptoms of tingling, numbness, and burning are common. Many people who have this condition just put up with it. Even if they consult their doctors for a diagnosis, there is no safe, effective drug treatment for it (sometimes calcium channel blockers are used).

Fortunately, Sally's internist knew that magnesium is the most effective treatment for both muscle cramps and Raynaud's because it improves circulation, stops spasms, and minimizes stress reactions. He put her on magnesium, 300 mg twice a day, and a daily multiple vitamin and mineral; after two months he added calcium, 500 mg twice a day.

It took three months for the Raynaud's to respond, but Sally couldn't believe how good she felt in the meantime. The muscle cramps improved within a week, and symptoms that she had thought were just part of getting old dramatically improved. Her energy increased as she was able to sleep better. Her bowel movements were also more regular, and she was much calmer than she had been in a long time.

Nutritional recommendations for Raynaud's include

liver-cleansing foods such as beets, dandelion greens, burdock root, and lemons, and foods rich in magnesium, including nuts, seeds, green vegetables, and whole grains. Foods to avoid or reduce to lessen the symptoms of Raynaud's syndrome include meat, alcohol, spices, and fatty, rich, fried, or salty foods.

TREATMENT FOR RAYNAUD'S

Magnesium: 300 mg twice per day

Calcium: 500 mg twice per day

Vitamin E as mixed tocopherols: 800 IU

Evening primrose oil: 6 capsules per day

Vitamin B_3: 100 mg three times a day (this vitamin sometimes causes the body to flush, as it increases circulation to the extremities)

Quercetin (a bioflavonoid): 500 mg per day

MAGNESIUM AND MUSCLE PAIN

A patient came for a consultation and wanted a total body X ray because she was having such severe episodes of pain—her whole body would go into spasm—that she thought she must have cancer. I asked her to try taking 300 mg of magnesium three times a day. Within three days she no longer had the spasms, and after three weeks she was free of pain.

**THREE THINGS YOU NEED TO KNOW ABOUT
MAGNESIUM AND MUSCLE PAIN**

1. Magnesium helps muscles relax.
2. Magnesium eliminates spasms.
3. Magnesium relaxes blood vessels in the fingers to treat
   Raynaud's syndrome.

Although this patient did not have cancer, research has shown that even the pain of cancer can respond to magnesium. Cancer sometimes metastasizes into nerve bundles located in the neck or lower back and may not respond to even the strongest analgesics such as morphine. There is a special receptor site called NMDA that is responsible for creating this type of nerve pain; magnesium blocks this receptor. In cases of severe pain, intravenous magnesium has shown very powerful analgesic effects.[15]

MAGNESIUM AND EXERCISE

Cells use energy packets called ATP (adenosine triphosphate), which are formed under the influence of magnesium. Some of the first studies showing the relationship between magnesium and physical performance were done on animals and found that decreased exercise capacity can be an early sign of magnesium deficiency. When the animals were given

THREE THINGS YOU NEED TO KNOW
ABOUT MAGNESIUM AND EXERCISE

1. Magnesium reduces lactic acid, which causes post-exercise pain.
2. Magnesium is lost during exercise.
3. Magnesium deficiency may cause sudden cardiac death in healthy athletes.

magnesium dissolved in water, their endurance was restored. Most human studies also confirm that both brief and extended exercise deplete magnesium.

One of the most amazing effects of magnesium on the neuromuscular system is that it provides more energy, even though the mineral generally acts as a relaxant and not a stimulant. If you are magnesium-deficient, your energy level will be low because you aren't producing the necessary energy to run your body. When you start taking magnesium, your energy level goes up. Magnesium's interactions with calcium help keep calcium from causing excessive muscle contraction. Excess calcium causes tension and tightness in all the muscles of the body, but when you take a balancing amount of magnesium, this tension releases within hours, days, or weeks, depending on the underlying level of magnesium deficiency in your body.

Exercise is often prescribed therapeutically for anxiety

and depression—to burn off steam (so to speak), to increase the circulation, and to get adrenaline pumping. Magnesium allows the body to burn fuel and create energy in an efficient cycle during exercise that does not lead to lactic acid production and buildup. For some individuals who exercise excessively or suffer from chronic fatigue syndrome, painful amounts of lactic acid build up in their muscles making exercise an unpleasant experience. Exercise itself places stress on your body, to which your adrenal glands respond by pumping out adrenaline, which interacts and binds to cell membranes in the presence of adequate magnesium.

Heavy exercisers, especially long-distance runners, can build up lactic acid and suffer shin splints and painful muscles, but they keep on running because they may be addicted to the adrenaline rush they get when they reach "the wall" in their workout. The wall feels like something you just can't break through, but you keep on pushing, and suddenly you get a burst of adrenaline and you're flying. That's the power of your adrenal glands when pushed to the maximum. Yet that stress-induced high is followed by a crash, when you don't repair the damage to your adrenal glands with good nutrition and restore the magnesium that was lost during exercise.

Many studies have shown that magnesium supplementation enhances the performance and endurance of long-distance runners, cross-country skiers, cyclists, and swimmers. It also reduces lactic acid buildup and postexercise cramps and pain. Since athletes undergo severe physical stress as well as the psychological drive to win, and most ingest suboptimal amounts of magnesium, they are vulnerable to magnesium deficiency.[16]

Years ago the coach of a Florida high school football team was concerned about his players' frequent complaints of leg cramps, so he gave them a calcium supplement on a very hot day before a rigorous game. Early in the second half, eleven players became disoriented and had difficulty walking. Their speech was slurred, they complained of muscle spasms, and they were breathing very deeply. Within an hour, eight of the boys collapsed into full-blown seizures; two had repeated seizures. Those having the worst symptoms had been playing the hardest. Thirteen more players reported headaches, blurred vision, muscle twitching, nausea, and weakness.[17] Eventually all the boys recovered, but what happened to create such a frightening scene in this group of healthy young men? Consider the facts. Those that were affected had all eaten a pre-game magnesium-deficient fast-food meal consisting mainly of carbohydrates and fats, and sodas containing phosphoric acid. With the increased magnesium loss from excessive sweating plus the calcium supplement, their magnesium stores had been driven dangerously low.[18]

Magnesium deficiency may also play a role in sudden cardiac death syndrome, which can affect athletes.[19] In a study of young, healthy, well-conditioned men, strenuous effort was reported to give rise to persistent magnesium deficiency and a related long-term increase in cholesterol, triglycerides, and blood sugar. This study postulates that the sudden death of athletes and other intensely training individuals during extreme exertion is triggered by the detrimental effects of persistent magnesium deficiency on the cardiovascular system.[20,21]

MAGNESIUM SUPPLEMENTS FOR EXERCISERS AND ATHLETES

Dr. Seelig, an internationally recognized magnesium specialist, recommends that athletes in training obtain at least 6–10 mg/kg/day (or 2.7–4.5 mg/lb/day) of magnesium to help replace the losses from exertion, sweating, and stress.

For a 220-pound man:	600–1,000 mg per day
For a 150-pound woman:	400–680 mg per day

These doses can be cut by 150 mg for people who exercise moderately (one to two hours a day).

CHAPTER 4

Migraines, Strokes, Head Injury, and Brain Surgery

THREE THINGS YOU NEED TO KNOW
ABOUT MAGNESIUM AND THE BRAIN

1. Magnesium protects the brain from the toxic effects of chemicals such as food additives.
2. Magnesium is a blood thinner, keeping thickened blood and tiny clots from causing blood vessel spasms and pain.
3. Magnesium relaxes head and neck muscle tension that makes migraines worse.

Martha knew that a migraine was looming when the sparks and wavy lines appeared before her eyes. Working became impossible, and she knew she would be looking at the loss of at least one day to a severe migraine attack. Medications such as codeine and ergotamine had not helped her over the years, instead making her feel drugged and tired after the headache finally passed. And the fancy new drugs Imitrex, Depakote, and Midrin did nothing for her head pain but did give her chest pain and make her more sick to her stomach. All Martha could do was lie in a darkened room with a cool cloth over her eyes, too nauseous to eat. This time, however, instead of trying to keep hydrated with lots of diet soda, as she usually did, she was going to drink mineral water with lemon and natural fruit juice.

Martha's daughter Mary, a nurse, had told her that aspartame, the sweetener in diet soda, causes headaches. Even though Martha loved her diet pop, drinking two liters a day on average, she knew she had to try to stop these headaches, both the daily ones and the one or two migraines a week.

Over the next few days, Martha's skin itched and she was nauseous, dizzy, and depressed. She thought she was having a hangover reaction to the medication she had taken for her migraine, but Mary told her she was going through aspartame withdrawal. She was also having strong cravings for her diet soda, but Mary insisted that she stay off it. Mary did some research on aspartame and how to cope with withdrawal and brought her mother a bottle of magnesium oxide supplements. The 500 mg twice a day seemed to help right away. By the next week, Martha's head felt clearer; she was more alert and less achy. She hadn't even realized that her joints and muscles had been tight and sore until she no longer had the symptoms. To her great relief, two weeks after eliminating aspartame from her diet, she realized that she hadn't had one of those headaches that she used to get daily. After two months of strictly avoiding aspartame, she still had no more headaches or migraines, except once after she had eaten something she had not known contained artificial sweetener. That convinced her even more that, for her, aspartame was poison.

ASPARTAME AND MSG: EXCITOTOXINS

Aspartame is, in fact, an excitotoxin, one of a group of substances, usually acidic amino acids, that in high amounts react with specialized receptors in the brain, causing destruction of certain types of neurons.

A growing number of neurosurgeons and neurologists are convinced that excitotoxins play a critical role in the development of several neurological disorders, including migraines, seizures, learning disorders in children, and neurodegenerative disorders such as Alzheimer's disease, Parkinson's disease, Huntington's disease, and amyotrophic lateral sclerosis (ALS).[1] Glutamate and aspartate are two important amino acids that act as neurotransmitters in the brain in very small concentrations, but they are also commonly available in food additives. Glutamate is in MSG, a flavor enhancer, and in hydrolyzed vegetable protein, found in hundreds of processed foods. Aspartate is one of three components of aspartame (NutraSweet, Equal), a sugar substitute. In higher concentrations as food additives, these chemicals constantly stimulate brain cells and can cause them to undergo a process of cell death known as excitotoxicity; the cells are excited to death.

HYPOGLYCEMIA

The brain becomes extremely vulnerable to excitotoxins during episodes of low blood sugar or hypoglycemia. Pound for pound, the brain uses more blood sugar than any other part of the body. Low blood sugar occurs in malnourished people and when people skip meals. It also occurs in individuals whose adrenal glands are depleted and can't mount the necessary adrenaline response to raise blood sugar when it gets too low. Magnesium is responsible for balancing blood sugar. With sufficient magnesium and balanced meals to prevent low blood sugar, you can protect yourself against headaches, attention deficit hyperactivity disorder, mood disorders, and even premenstrual tension. Supporting the brain as much as possible with safe nutrients and a safe environment, you may never need the brain-altering medications that are prescribed for these disorders.

Medically, hypoglycemia occurs when blood sugar (glucose) drops to a low of 50 mg/dl (normal is about 80–110 mg/dl). If you eat a highly refined diet with lots of white sugar and white flour, foods whose carbohydrates are rapidly absorbed into the bloodstream, your blood sugar will quickly become elevated; when it reaches a certain maximum, insulin enters the bloodstream and quickly ushers the excess glucose away into the cells of the body, causing your blood sugar to drop. The more sugar you eat and absorb, the more insulin is released and the quicker your blood sugar can fall. This abrupt drop causes adrenaline to be released from the adrenal glands to make sure that the blood sugar does not fall so low that you faint. When that adrenaline mobilizes the sugar stores in the liver to elevate your blood sugar, however, it also produces a fight-or-flight reaction, which may give you a sense of anxiety or impending doom. It may even feel like a panic attack because you don't equate your symptoms with low blood sugar. At this point, if you eat something to pick you up or comfort you, such as a candy bar or an aspartame-containing diet drink, or if you are exposed to other environmental toxins, your glucose-deprived, magnesium-deficient brain will be more vulnerable to the effects of the excitotoxins. Many diseases of the nervous system are being associated with excitotoxin buildup in the brain, including migraines, seizures, strokes, and brain injury.

If you have magnesium deficiency and regularly use aspartame, the toxicity is magnified and can result in headaches and migraines. You can easily identify whether your headaches are caused by aspartame: Give yourself sixty days without any aspartame and judge for yourself. And if you want to minimize the withdrawal effects, take 150 mg of elemental magnesium three to four times a day (see page 71 for more on dosages).

Magnesium helps prevent the chain of events that causes cell death due to low blood sugar and exposure to other toxins besides excitotoxins. One of the most important neuroprotectants known, magnesium helps defend our cells against potential neurotoxins in our environment, such as pesticides, herbicides, food additives, solvents, and cleaning products.[2] Drs. Michael and Mary Dan Eades, authors of *Protein Power*, state that if they had only one supplement to give their patients, they would choose magnesium above all others.[3] In Chapter 10 we will talk more about the myriad toxins to which we are subjected on a daily basis, how we can avoid them, and how magnesium can protect us from harm.

MIGRAINE MECHANISMS

Twenty-five million Americans suffer from migraines. Statistically, women have more migraines than men, especially in the twenty-to-fifty age group. The following biochemical events involving low magnesium have been identified in migraine sufferers and may set the stage for migraines.[4]

- In nonmenopausal women, estrogen rises before the period, causing a shift of blood magnesium into bone and muscles. As a result, magnesium levels in the brain are lowered.
- When magnesium is low, it is unable to do its job to counteract the clotting action of calcium on the blood. Tiny blood clots are said to clog up tiny brain

blood vessels, leading to migraines. Several other substances that help create blood clots are increased when magnesium is too low.
- Low brain magnesium promotes neurotransmitter hyperactivity and nerve excitation that can lead to headaches.

Several conditions that trigger migraines are also associated with magnesium deficiency, including pregnancy, alcohol intake, usage of some diuretic drugs, stress, and menstruation. Magnesium deficiency is related to migraines in so many ways.

- Magnesium relaxes blood vessels and allows them to dilate, reducing the spasms and constrictions that can cause migraines.
- Magnesium regulates the action of brain neurotransmitters and inflammatory substances, which may play a role in migraines when unbalanced.
- Magnesium thins the blood, somewhat like aspirin, preventing the formation of tiny clots that can block blood vessels and cause pain.
- Magnesium relaxes muscles and prevents the buildup of lactic acid, which, along with muscle tension, can worsen head pain.

A group of three thousand patients given 200 mg of magnesium daily had an 80 percent reduction in their migraine symptoms.[5] This study did not have a control group, so the results could be questioned, but it aroused a lot of excitement and triggered a flurry of research on magnesium and migraines. A great deal of that research was done by Dr. Alexander Mauskop, director of the New York Headache Center, working with Drs. Bella and Burton Altura, who have been studying migraines and migraine treatments for about ten years. Their research team consistently found that magnesium is deficient in people with migraine and many other types of headache; treating the deficiency alleviates the headache.

Dr. Mauskop with the Drs. Altura undertook many studies using sensitive magnesium ion electrodes.[6] During one of the first they found a deficiency in magnesium ions but not total serum magnesium in migraine patients.[7] Migraine sufferers with low magnesium ion levels who were given intravenous magnesium experienced a complete alleviation of their symptoms, including sensitivity to light and sound.[8] Subsequent studies of migraine patients confirmed a common pattern and support a role for magnesium deficiency in the development of headaches.[9] The researchers found that infusion of magnesium resulted in a rapid and sustained relief of acute migraine. Because of an excellent safety profile and low cost, they recommend oral magnesium supplementation for migraine sufferers at a level of 6 mg/kg/day.[10]

Patients with cluster headaches, a very severe form of recurrent headache, have also been reported to have low magnesium ion levels. Some people suffer up to twenty bouts of pain daily in a siege that can last for months.

Another study from Altura, Altura, and Mauskop examined the possibility that patients with cluster headaches and low magnesium ion levels may respond to an intravenous infusion of magnesium sulfate. Within fifteen minutes of an intravenous dose of magnesium, nine patients with cluster headaches had their acute headache aborted.[11] Blood ionized magnesium testing thus proves to be useful in elucidating the pathogenesis of cluster headaches and in identifying patients who may benefit from treatment with magnesium, much as it does for migraines.[12]

Another research team treated eighty-one patients with ongoing migraine headaches with 300 mg of magnesium twice a day. The frequency of migraines was reduced by

---

MIGRAINE TREATMENT

Identify food allergies that may trigger migraines

Magnesium: 300 mg one to two times per day

Calcium: 500 mg twice per day

Vitamin B_2 (riboflavin): 400 mg per day

Vitamin B complex: 50 mg per day (it is necessary to take the complex to prevent imbalances if you are taking large amounts of one B vitamin)

Feverfew (*Tanacetum parthenium*): 100 mg per day

Stress therapies

Regular exercise

Aspirin has been used to treat headaches for decades. Magnesium-buffered aspirin, however, is preferred by heavy users. Could magnesium be responsible for some of its beneficial effects? The same question applies to buffered aspirin used in heart disease.

41.6 percent in the magnesium group but by only 15.8 percent in a control group that received placebos. The number of migraine days and drug consumption for pain also decreased significantly in the magnesium group. High-dose oral magnesium appears to be effective in migraine treatment and prevention.[13]

In Dr. Mauskop's *What Your Doctor May Not Tell You About Migraines* he outlines his "triple therapy" for migraines. It includes magnesium, vitamin B$_2$ (riboflavin), and a well-known migraine herb, feverfew.

HEAD INJURY, BRAIN SURGERY, AND STROKE

Magnesium does much more than any drug to protect the blood circulation and the brain:

- It's a vasodilator, opening up blood vessels.
- It protects the endothelium, or inner layer of blood vessels.

- It closes the calcium channel to excessive calcium influx.

MAGNESIUM-DEFICIENT BRAINS

With most of the U.S. population deficient in magnesium,[14] many Americans are at greater risk for a host of serious problems, including stroke with severe poststroke complications, depending on the degree of magnesium deficiency; poor recovery from head injury with escalating neurological damage; neurotoxin damage from vast numbers of chemicals in our air, food, and water: seizure disorders; Alzheimer's disease; and Parkinson's disease.[15] These conditions are the neurological equivalent of heart disease. After all, both heart and brain are excitable tissues that give off electrical energy, and both must have magnesium. The complexity of the mechanisms of central nervous system hyperexcitability due to magnesium deficiency is only now being appreciated.[16]

HEAD INJURY AND MAGNESIUM

Traumatic brain injury (TBI) is a major public health problem throughout the world. There are more than four hundred thousand patients with TBI in the United States alone. From animal studies, we know that brain magnesium levels fall dramatically at the site of injury as this mineral is depleted in a cascade of events.[17] In sixty-six human subjects with acute blunt head trauma, the greater the degree of injury, the greater the calcium-ion-to-magnesium-ion ratio.

Such findings provide evidence of magnesium ion changes in blood after traumatic brain injury, which could be of both diagnostic and prognostic value.[18] Studies of both animals and brain trauma victims suggest that higher magnesium levels are associated with a better recovery.[19] Giving sufficient magnesium will create a better healing outcome. Magnesium sulfate significantly reduces brain edema following brain injury and is used to treat patients with severe TBI without adverse effects.[20] This is crucial information to give your doctor if your child suffers a head injury or any family member is involved in a motor vehicle accident.

Ionic magnesium testing makes the diagnosis of posttraumatic headaches much easier. Abnormalities in magnesium ion concentration and the calcium-ion-to-magnesium-ion ratio were found in children with posttraumatic headaches, but total serum magnesium levels were normal.[21] Obviously, studies using only the total serum magnesium test would miss the diagnosis and fail to properly treat these patients. (See Chapter 12 for a full discussion of magnesium testing.)

A magnesium deficit from head injury is slow to reverse. According to Dr. Blaylock magnesium takes thirty minutes to get into the spinal fluid, three hours to reach the cortical area directly under the skull, and a full four to six hours to reach the deep brain tissues. Experiments with Navy Seals and marathon runners show that after a month of intensive training, they experience magnesium deficiency and, if no supplements are taken, the deficiency is still present three to six months later. It only makes sense that if your diet is deficient and you're under stress, physical or emotional, you need to replace your magnesium stores daily.

BRAIN INJURY, ALCOHOL, AND MAGNESIUM

Drs. Bella and Burton Altura discuss the direct cause-and-effect relationship between alcohol-induced headache and risk of brain injury and stroke.[22] They note that binge drinking of alcohol is associated with an ever-growing number of strokes and cases of sudden death, with alcohol causing vasospasm and rupture of the cerebral arteries.[23] In animal studies, high doses of alcohol caused a rapid fall in levels of magnesium ions in the brain and an elevation of calcium, followed by cerebral vessel spasm and rupture of cerebral blood vessels (stroke).[24,25] In human studies, people with mild head injury have been found to exhibit early deficits in magnesium ions; the greater the degree of head injury, the greater and more profound the deficit in magnesium ions, and the greater the level of calcium ions compared to magnesium ions. Patients with histories of alcohol abuse or ingestion of alcohol prior to head injury exhibited greater deficits in magnesium ions (and higher calcium-ion-to-magnesium-ion ratios) and, unlike the subjects without alcohol, remained in the hospital at least several days longer. Data on 105 men and women with different types of stroke indicate that, on average, a 20 percent deficit in magnesium ions is seen, while total serum magnesium is usually normal.[26]

The Alturas also report that in other human studies, it has been shown that migraines, headache, dizziness, and hangover, which accompany ethanol ingestion, are associated with rapid deficits in magnesium ion level but not in total serum magnesium, which obscures the diagnosis if only total serum magnesium is measured. And since magnesium is necessary to regulate calcium, its deficiency creates calcium-induced vascular spasms and pathology.[27] Migraines and alcohol-associated headaches can be treated with intravenous administration of magnesium sulfate.[28] Premenstrual tension headache and its exacerbation by alcohol in women is also accompanied by deficits in magnesium ions and elevation in the calcium-ion-to-magnesium-ion ratio. Intravenous magnesium sulfate corrects both the premenstrual tension headache and the serum deficit in magnesium ions.

Animal experiments show that intravenous magnesium can prevent alcohol-induced hemorrhagic stroke and the subsequent fall in brain magnesium ion level as well as other metabolic factors.[29] Recent data indicate that alcohol-induced cellular loss of magnesium ions is associated with cellular calcium overload and generation of free radicals; however, pretreatment with vitamin E can also prevent alcohol-induced vascular injury and pathology in the brain.[30] (Learn more about free radicals on page 193.)

BRAIN SURGERY AND MAGNESIUM

During and after brain surgery, magnesium's many attributes come into play by preventing stroke, keeping calcium from entering damaged cells, and decreasing the incidence of seizure and spasm. These favorable effects have all been proven unequivocally in animal studies, but clinical experience in the neurosurgical operating room also proves its efficacy as lives are being saved. Many surgeons make it standard procedure to administer intravenous magnesium to all their surgical patients before an operation. Dr. Bernard Horn, a general surgeon in California, has given intravenous magnesium sulfate to more than eight thousand patients over a fifteen-year period. Dr. Horn reports that patients' blood pressures as high as 200 over 150 would normalize before surgery.[31]

Intravenous magnesium sulfate also acts as a general anesthetic so that during surgery the dose of other chemical anesthetics can be safely reduced. Using intravenous magnesium also results in lower postoperative pain scores, less pain medication needed in the twenty-four hours after surgery, and less postoperative nausea and vomiting. Magnesium sulfate is therefore a safe and cost-effective addition to such general anesthetics as propofol, remifentanil, and mivacurium.[32]

STROKE

All deaths due to stroke among Taiwan residents (17,133 cases) from 1989 through 1993 were compared with deaths from other causes (17,133 controls). It was determined that the higher the magnesium levels in water, the lower the incidence of stroke.[33]

THREE THINGS YOU NEED TO KNOW ABOUT MAGNESIUM AND BRAIN SURGERY

1. Good neurosurgeons give magnesium to all their surgical patients.
2. Magnesium helps the brain recover from head injury.
3. Magnesium can prevent strokes or make them less damaging.

Decades of research show that withdrawal of magnesium from cerebral arteries causes them to spasm, whereas elevated magnesium produces relaxation.[34,35,36] Animal studies show that when there is normal or elevated magnesium in the brain, the damage caused by stroke is reduced and the neurological deficit is lessened. This is because magnesium blocks calcium from flooding the cells and causing injury. Further research indicates that the area of the brain damaged by stroke contains injured neurons that remain hyperactive for several hours after the stroke has occurred.[37] These cells are frantically struggling to survive and need even more oxygen, glucose, and magnesium than normal. In addition, when these vital nutrients are deficient, those neurons become especially vulnerable to the damaging effects of excitotoxins that rush in to fill the void left by escaping nutrients. Hospitalized patients commonly have low magnesium levels, which means that neurons are even less likely to survive. According to one researcher, a state of severe magnesium deficiency alone is enough for rats to develop widespread injury to their brains.[38]

A study of stroke patients in New York highlights the absolute requirement for magnesium intervention in the ER. Ninety-eight patients admitted to the emergency rooms of three hospitals with a diagnosis of stroke exhibited early and significant deficits in magnesium ions as measured with a sensitive ion-selective electrode. The stroke patients also demonstrated a high calcium-ion-to-magnesium-ion ratio, signs of increased vascular tone and cerebral vessel spasm.[39]

DIURETICS DRY OUT THE BRAIN

An elderly woman's total serum magnesium level became depleted due to a diuretic she was taking for hypertension.[40] She was admitted to the hospital with severe weakness and developed an overt psychosis with paranoid delusions. Fortunately, her deficiency was identified, and following large intravenous doses of magnesium, her symptoms disappeared within twenty-four hours. She was unable to discontinue magnesium therapy without a recurrence of her symptoms as long as she was taking the diuretic. No other abnormalities were found to explain her condition. People who are prescribed diuretics should check with their doctor about taking at least 600 mg a day of supplemental magnesium in divided doses.

MAGNESIUM AND SEIZURES

The brain is in a state of constant electrical activity. Brain cells are either stimulating or suppressing activity in a delicate push-and-pull balance. These cells are like switches: some switches are turned on and some are turned off by neurotransmitter chemicals. The action of these neurotransmitters could not take place without calcium, magnesium, and zinc, which play various roles in switching on and off the nerve cells to electrical stimulation.

Brain cells altered by trauma, chemicals, or severe stress can be permanently switched on and fire excessively. Repeated firing in many nerve cells may result in seizures. Magnesium raises the threshold for seizures, reducing the chance of them developing at all. Conversely, experimental studies have shown that low magnesium in the body significantly lowers the threshold for seizures, that is, makes them more likely to occur.[41]

Hypertension, High Cholesterol, Spastic Heart, Angina, Arrhythmia, Arteriosclerosis, and Heart Attack

THREE THINGS YOU NEED TO KNOW ABOUT MAGNESIUM AND HEART DISEASE

1. Magnesium prevents muscle spasms of the heart blood vessels, which can lead to heart attack.
2. Magnesium prevents muscle spasms of the peripheral blood vessels, which can lead to high blood pressure.
3. Magnesium prevents calcium buildup in cholesterol plaque in arteries, which leads to clogged arteries.

Annette was tired of people's shocked reaction when they learned that she was recovering from a heart attack. She knew that the common image of heart disease was that it targeted aggressive, overweight men who smoked and ate too much. Annette, on the other hand, was slim, reserved, and a vegetarian who ate a low-fat diet. She chuckled when friends tried to tell her about the Dr. Dean Ornish vegetarian diet for reversing heart disease, because she'd lived according to that diet.

She was only fifty-six, a nonsmoker, with exemplary cholesterol, but she did have slightly elevated blood pressure, her only risk factor. Yet she had had a mild heart attack. Now she suffered from daily palpitations and was on several medications that seemed to drain her energy more with every passing day. She was also simply too afraid to exert herself for fear of bringing on another heart attack.

Annette was becoming an invalid, and at her next appointment her cardiologist was shocked at her worn-out appearance. He decided to run some blood tests and was urged by a student doctor to order the new ionized magnesium test. The results of that test were so low that the lab rushed the results to him the next morning. His nurse immediately called Annette to come in, saying the doctor had found something that would help her feel better. Annette was prescribed a magnesium preparation that she mixed with water (Slow-Mag) that began to work within twenty-four hours. She was amazed that her muscle aches, insomnia, palpitations, and fatigue all but disappeared. She was even able to cut back on her other medications. Her doctor vowed to test all his patients' magnesium ion levels from then on, and wondered aloud if it had been

AN IMPORTANT REMINDER ABOUT TAKING MAGNESIUM WITH PRESCRIPTION DRUGS

You may experience a decreased need for your drugs as magnesium deficiency is corrected or as magnesium treats your symptoms or reverses your condition. In other words, the symptoms for which the drug was prescribed may clear up due to the magnesium, making the drug unnecessary or toxic and causing new symptoms. Patients and doctors should be on the alert for a shift in symptoms. Be sure to work with your doctor to lower your medication doses safely.

low magnesium in the first place that had led to Annette's heart attack.

As we will learn in Chapter 7, obstetricians are quite familiar with the use of magnesium for hypertension in women about to deliver. Unfortunately, they aren't talking to cardiologists or even to family doctors about the importance of magnesium in treating general hypertension, one of the main risk factors for heart disease.

Heart disease is the number one killer of both American women and men, accounting for half of all U.S. deaths (52.3 percent of the total deaths occurring in women compared to 47.7 percent in men). According to the American Heart Association, every thirty-three seconds someone in the United States dies of cardiovascular disease; that's approaching one million deaths annually. Hypertension occurs in fifty million Americans and accounts for an estimated 29.3 million office visits a year to allopathic doctors (M.D.'s)[1] Antihypertensive drug prescriptions are given at most of these appointments, even though magnesium has been used successfully for over half a century by medical doctors, osteopaths, and naturopathic doctors.[2,3]

THE SLIPPERY ROAD TO HEART ATTACK

STEP ONE: LOSS OF ARTERIAL ELASTICITY

The coronary arteries bringing oxygen-filled blood from inside the heart through the aorta to the heart muscle are very, very small, only about 3 mm across (a nickel is 2 mm thick). It doesn't take much to plug them up with a tiny blood clot or to imagine them collapsing when in spasm. Magnesium prevents blood clot formation and artery spasm. These coronary arteries get even smaller as they split into two, then four, then eight and so on as they descend toward the bottom of the heart. Each of these splits is called a bifurcation. According to cardiologists, about 85 percent of sclerotic plaques initially form near bifurcations. It is widely believed that the development of these plaques is a response to injury. This means that something, such as an infection, may be damaging the arteries, rather than just fat and calcium building up like silt in a river.

Endothelial cells are a single layer of specialized cells that form the inside membrane of an artery. The subendothelial layer (the next layer in) is a very thin connective tissue that contains elastin. As its name implies, this is the layer responsible for providing much of the elasticity in your arteries. It is important to note that your body requires magnesium to maintain healthy elastin.

Smooth muscle cells are the next layer. Smooth muscle cells provide integrity and control the dilation of the arterial cavity, triggered by the calcium/magnesium ratio in the body. Calcium causes contraction and magnesium causes relaxation, which together control the blood pressure and flow in the artery. A final messenger for the dilation response is nitric oxide, which is dependent on magnesium.

One of the earliest signs of magnesium deficiency is degeneration of elastin in the subendothelium. Animals on low-magnesium diets lose the elasticity of their arterial system. Coronary arteries require even more elasticity than other arteries because they must stretch and flex as the heart expands and contracts. Loss of elasticity results in inflammation of the endothelial and subendothelial layers at points that are most mechanically challenged by stretching the bifurcations. Imagine a small rubber-band-like tube shaped like a Y. In your mind's eye-grasp the two legs of the Y in one hand. With your other hand, grip the single leg. Begin pulling them apart just as though they were stretching on the surface of the heart. Stretch it as far as you can. Where is the shape weakest? If we left the rubber tube out in the sun for a week or so, what would happen if you slowly stretched it again? Where might you expect the first crack to appear? Most of the time it would happen at or near where one tube becomes two—at the bifurcation. If your artery loses elasticity, it makes sense that the problem might show up at or near the bifurcation.

STEP TWO: THE INFLAMMATORY RESPONSE

Inflammation begins with injury of the artery wall, leading to white blood cells and cholesterol hovering around trying to heal the damage. At this stage in the process, if there is too much calcium and not enough magnesium in the bloodstream, excess calcium precipitates around the area of inflammation in the artery wall. The area becomes rigid and interferes with blood flow.

STEP THREE: HEART ATTACK

Over time, the above steps weaken and plug the coronary arteries and slowly kill small areas of the heart muscle. The final result is severe chest pain, damage to a larger portion of heart muscle, and heart attack.[4]

Some of the first evidence for the use of magnesium against heart disease came from epidemiological studies in Wales, Taiwan, Sweden, Finland, and Japan showing that death rates from coronary heart disease are higher in communities with magnesium-deficient water and magnesium-deficient diets.[5] Areas where calcium in the water is much higher than magnesium or where dietary intake of calcium is higher than magnesium showed even more coronary heart disease. A U.S. study done over a seven-year period followed fourteen thousand men and women and concluded that low magnesium in the diet may contribute to the origin of coronary atherosclerosis and acute heart attack.[6]

The Centers for Disease Control and Prevention in Atlanta followed twelve thousand people for nineteen years, at the end of which 4,282 people had died, 1,005 from heart disease. Risk of dying from heart disease was highest in those with magnesium deficiency. Researchers made a conservative estimate that 11 percent of the half a million people dying of heart disease in 1993 could have been directly related to magnesium deficiency.[7] If more accurate measurements for magnesium deficiency were used, such as ionic magnesium testing, we would find the numbers to be even higher and the need for magnesium even greater.

The evidence has been mounting for decades that magnesium plays a crucial role in the prevention of both atherosclerosis and arteriosclerosis.[8,9] It maintains the elasticity of the artery wall, dilates blood vessels, prevents calcium deposits, and is necessary for the maintenance of healthy muscles, including the heart muscle itself. For all these reasons, magnesium is critical to the maintenance of a healthy heart.[10] One of the pivotal metabolic chemicals in the body is nitric oxide (NO). It is a very simple compound made from nitrogen and oxygen, but it packs a powerful punch. Nitric oxide controls vasodilation, but this activity is under the direction of magnesium.[11]

HIGH CHOLESTEROL

The upper limit of normal cholesterol is 200 mg/dl, but it appears that over time, with the average cholesterol in the general population becoming more elevated, the values that medicine accepts as normal have risen. Some doctors are taking a stand and revising the upper limit of normal down to 180 mg/dl. As with hypertension, the actual cause of most cases of high cholesterol is said to be unknown. High cholesterol tends to run in families and occurs in association with low thyroid hormone production or hypothyroidism, liver disease, and pregnancy.

There are several types of cholesterol with different functions, some of which we label good and some bad. Cholesterol associated with high-density lipoprotein, HDL, is generally considered to be beneficial to the body. It apparently functions to remove other cholesterol or fatty deposits from blood vessel walls and the blood itself, bringing it to the liver for processing and excretion. Low-density lipoprotein, LDL, is commonly thought to be harmful to the body because it carries cholesterol into the bloodstream, promoting the buildup of cholesterol plaque on the arterial walls. Very-low-density lipoproteins, VLDLs, are made into LDLs in the liver and are also thought to be harmful.

But all of these cholesterols are normally found in the body. What's *not* normal is the high amounts of oxidized cholesterol (cholesterol abnormally bound with oxygen) that we eat in processed foods, fast foods, and fried foods. In addition, chlorine, fluoride in water, pesticides, and other environmental pollutants can also oxidize cholesterol in the body. It is this oxidized cholesterol that researchers are concerned about when it comes to heart disease.[12] Regular use of antioxidants such as magnesium, vitamin E, vitamin A, vitamin C, and green tea can lower oxidized cholesterol levels. There is compelling evidence that magnesium therapy reduces cholesterol levels,[13,14,15] even when there is a genetic risk factor present for hypercholesterolemia.[16]

There are no visible symptoms of high cholesterol beyond the associated signs of a bad diet, sedentary lifestyle, smoking, alcohol intake, and stress. A poor diet with a high intake of saturated and polyunsaturated fats, hydrogenated oils, fried foods, meat, sugar, coffee, and alcohol will elevate cholesterol levels, especially when a person lacks fiber from whole grains and vegetables. Add a sedentary lifestyle, and cholesterol increases. The very diet that promotes elevated cholesterol also causes magnesium deficiency. Unfortunately, many doctors do not have the time or inclination to educate patients about correct eating habits that could reduce their cholesterol, instead using medication to treat the problem. To be fair, many patients don't have the inclination to comply even if their doctor recommends a diet, exercise, and weight loss. Adding magnesium supplementation to lifestyle changes, however, gives patients more dramatic improvement, making compliance easier.

Many of us have been conditioned to believe that elevated cholesterol is the only cause of heart disease; that is why marketers have been so successful in getting us to replace the saturated fat of butter with hydrogenated vegetable oils. Yet epidemiologists and dental anthropologists proved long ago that various world cultures that ate high-cholesterol diets for thousands of years (including meat, lard, cream, butter, and eggs) suffered very little, if any, heart disease.[17] Almost all the long-lived, healthy communities where degenerative disease and heart disease were unknown included significant amounts of natural, unprocessed meat or dairy in their diets. And it is also clear that once a country is exposed to refined and processed food, or

A major disadvantage of low-fat products is that they contain extra sugar in order to capture the taste buds. Even worse is aspartame, a synthetic sweetener with a daunting list of ninety-two side effects to its name. To maintain your health, avoid both.

"altered" meat and "altered" dairy, health declines in a number of ways.[18,19,20] Hydrogenated oils are unsaturated oils and for that reason were thought to be healthier than saturated fats such as butter. But the processing of liquid vegetable oil by heat, pressure, and chemicals to change it into a solid fat creates an unhealthy synthetic product called a trans fatty acid (as opposed to the natural cis fatty acid). Only in the late 1990s did we find out that these highly refined hydrogenated oils themselves promote atherosclerotic plaque much more than butter. In fact, some scientists say that the rise of myocardial infarctions, and heart disease in general, can be traced back to the 1930s, when hydrogenated oils were first introduced. We now know that trans fatty acids cause arterial damage and cancer. Be sure to read labels to avoid this substance.

HOMOCYSTEINURIA

Dr. Kilmer McCully was the first researcher, back in 1969, to identify a condition of increased levels of an amino acid, homocysteine, in the urine of patients with heart disease, which could be reversed with certain nutrients.[21,22] Homocysteine is a normal by-product of protein digestion, which in elevated amounts causes oxidized cholesterol, which damages blood vessels. (See page 89 for a definition of oxidized cholesterol.) For certain individuals who lack specific enzymes for protein digestion, homocysteine can become a real problem.

NORMAL LIPID VALUES

Cholesterol: 180 mg/dl

HDL cholesterol: greater than 45 mg/dl

LDL cholesterol: less than 130 mg/dl

VLDL cholesterol: less than 35 mg/dl

Total-cholesterol-to-HDL ratio: in men the optimal ratio is less than 3.43 (average = 4.97); in women the optimal ratio is less than 3.27 (average = 4.44)

A healthy level of homocysteine is below 12 micromoles per liter of blood (12 μmol/L). Homocysteine levels greater than 12 μmol/L are considered high. Twenty to 40 percent of the general population have elevated levels of homocysteine. Individuals with high levels have almost four times the risk of suffering a heart attack compared to people with normal levels.[23] Elevated homocysteine is high on the list of risk factors for heart disease and serves as an even stronger marker than high cholesterol for heart disease and blood clotting disorders.[24,25]

The more relevant marker, in my opinion, is low magnesium, since the major enzymes involved in homocysteine metabolism are magnesium-dependent.[26] McCully blames too much protein in the diet for elevated homocysteine. However, when magnesium, vitamin B_6, vitamin B_{12}, and folic acid are deficient, the body is not able to properly digest protein. The B vitamins were readily available in the typical diet a hundred years ago; now that they're absent from the diet, homocysteine becomes elevated and heart disease results. When these metabolic nutrients are reintroduced through diet or supplements, the high homocysteine levels are reversed and the symptoms of heart disease diminish. Ongoing research confirms that B_6, B_{12}, and folic acid together with magnesium are necessary to prevent blood vessel damage induced by high levels of homocysteine in the blood.[27] In short, the successful treatment of homocysteinemia relies on dietary changes that include B vitamins and magnesium.[28,29,30]

It must be remembered, however, that high homocysteine is also a marker for all causes of mortality and signifies that a deficiency in essential nutrients has a far-reaching effect on the body beyond heart disease.[31]

ATHEROSCLEROSIS

It is easy to confuse the terms *arteriosclerosis* and *atherosclerosis*; in fact, many people use them interchangeably. *Arteriosclerosis* is the overall term for sclerosis or scarring of the arteries. *Atherosclerosis* is scarring or thickening specifically due to fatty plaques. When the diameter of an artery is narrowed by fat deposits, a blood clot or an arterial spasm can be the final straw that results in angina, heart attack, or stroke. Complications of this preventable condition cause over a third of all deaths in the United States.

**SUPPLEMENT AND DRUG INTERACTIONS
IN HEART DISEASE**

1. Calcium interacts with verapamil (Calan, Isoptin, Vere-lan). This is a calcium channel blocker, and calcium interferes with the hypotensive effect of this drug. Avoid calcium until your doctor weans you off this drug.
2. Vitamin B_1 (thiamine) interacts with furosemide (Lasix). Lasix causes increased urinary excretion of B_1 so supplements of this vitamin may be necessary.
3. Vitamin B_6 interacts with hydralazine (Alazine, Apresazide, Apresoline, Unipres). Hydralazine causes increased excretion of vitamin B_6; supplements of the nutrient may be necessary.
4. Calcium, magnesium, and potassium interact with furosemide, which causes urinary excretion of these minerals. Monitor levels of these nutrients and replace as necessary.
5. Grapefruit juice makes felodipine and nifepidine (Adalat, Procardia) more powerful; it increases the action of these drugs by temporarily blocking the enzyme that clears them from the body. You may have to avoid grapefruit juice while on these medications.
6. Magnesium, calcium, potassium, and sodium interact with thiazide diuretics such as chlorthiazide (Diuril, Aldoril, Diachlor) and hydrochlorthiazide (Hydrodiuril).

Thiazides work by increasing urinary excretion of sodium, which presumably lowers blood pressure. However, significant amounts of calcium, potassium, and magnesium are also excreted. Magnesium at 600 mg per day may have to be increased to 900 mg if you are on thiazide diuretics or digitalis because both drugs cause excretion of magnesium. Your doctor should do an ionized magnesium test to determine your needs.

7. Potassium and magnesium deficiencies lead to arrhythmias in patients on digoxin (Lanoxin).

8. Small increases in plasma calcium increase digoxin (Lanoxin) toxicity. Some specialists advise avoiding high-calcium foods for two hours before and after taking this drug.

9. Calcium should be supplemented due to decreased absorption of vitamin D with patients using cholesterol-lowering drugs colestipol or cholestyramine.

10. Colestipol (Colestid) interferes with absorption of iron, folate, and vitamins A, D, E, and K.

11. Cholestyramine (Quesyran, Cholybar) interferes with absorption of iron, folate, and vitamins A, D, E, and K.

12. Heparin interferes with renal hydroxylation of vitamin D. This could lead to osteopenia; your doctor may need to check $1,25 (OH)_2 D_3$ cholecalciferol levels.

13. Vitamin K inactivates coumadin (Warfarin); coumadin interferes with vitamin K synthesis.[32]

Researchers have identified various causes of damage to the inner wall of arteries, including homocysteine, an amino acid discussed earlier; infection by an organism called chlamydia; distorted blood flow around the mound of fat; free radicals; high blood sugar; high blood pressure; and lack of oxygen. As described previously, the damaged tissue of the artery wall initiates an inflammatory process. The inflammation then attracts bad cholesterol (LDL) and calcium, which build up into a solid scar. Magnesium has a role to play in reducing homocysteine levels, preventing free radicals, balancing blood sugar, and reducing high blood pressure.

HYPERTENSION

Hypertension is an elevation of blood pressure suffered by more than fifty million Americans. Normal blood pressure is 120–140 over 80–90. Systolic pressure is the first number and relates to the pump pressure that the heart muscle creates to push blood into the arteries. Diastolic pressure is the second number and is the pressure that the arteries maintain when the heart is relaxed, or between heartbeats, to keep the arteries open. Hypertension is either primary or secondary. Primary hypertension has no single cause and occurs in 90 percent of all hypertensive patients. Secondary hypertension is secondary to another disease. Causes of primary hypertension include high cholesterol, family history, obesity, diet, smoking, stress, and excessive salt intake. Most often, hypertension is diagnosed during a routine physical exam. It presents no distinguishing signs or symptoms unless the condition is very advanced, in which case headache, dizziness, and blurred vision can occur.

In Western medicine, the first line of drug treatment for hypertension is typically the use of diuretics, or water pills. When patients are prescribed diuretics, they are warned that the most common side effect is a deficiency of potassium, which spills out in the urine. To prevent it, they are advised to eat bananas and oranges. What they are not told is that magnesium is drained out along with potassium. Recall that magnesium deficiency leads to blood vessels that are less relaxed and more susceptible to spasm and tension, a precursor to hypertension; thus the very treatment for hypertension worsens the problem.[33] (Ironically, replacing potassium doesn't help patients who are also magnesium-deficient, because the body is unable to deliver potassium to the cells without sufficient magnesium. Also, the so-called potassium-sparing diuretics still commonly deplete other minerals, including magnesium.)[34]

If blood pressure is not controlled with diuretics, the next choice may be ACE inhibitors, calcium channel blockers, antiadrenergic drugs, or vasodilators. One cardiologist confided to me that if a patient's blood pressure is still high after using five different antihypertensive drugs at one time, he then knows the problem is magnesium deficiency.

Fortunately, other cardiologists know that magnesium is a physiological necessity and a pharmacological treasure to use before pharmacological intervention. They call magnesium the ideal drug: It is safe, cheap, and simple to use, with a wide therapeutic range, a short half-life, and little or no tendency toward drug interactions.[35]

Even before drugs, diet is the first treatment of choice for hypertension. Research shows a direct relationship between the amount of magnesium in the diet and the ability to avoid high blood pressure.[36] The Alturas first demonstrated that diets deficient in magnesium will produce hypertension in experimental animals.[37] Diet may lower the blood pressure successfully due to a combination of weight loss and increased intake of the vitamin and mineral cofactors necessary in blood pressure control. For example, increased levels of minerals such as potassium and magnesium in the diet have a suppressive effect on calcium-regulating hormones, which influence blood pressure.[38] The arterial blood pressure appears to go up as the levels of magnesium ions and total serum magnesium go down.[39]

Note: Some forms of severe high blood pressure are hereditary or due to kidney disease and do require medication. Also, if the arteries in the body are damaged from long-term atherosclerotic injury and scarring, unfortunately they may no longer respond to magnesium and you may require medications to keep your blood pressure under control.

ANGINA

Angina describes an episodic pain in the region of the chest and/or down the left arm, due to lack of oxygen to the heart muscle and a buildup of carbon dioxide and other metabolites. Usually the pain, which can be a mild ache, pressure, or fullness, or a crushing blow, comes on with exercise (especially in the cold), emotional stress, a heavy meal, or even a vivid dream, and is relieved (within five minutes) by rest and nitroglycerine.

The lack of sufficient blood flow carrying life-giving oxygen and nutrients can be due to blocked coronary arteries or spasms in these tiny vessels. Angina is labeled "unstable" when symptoms become more severe; unstable angina implies a greater risk for heart attack. Another type of angina is called Prinzmetal's, which is angina that occurs at rest, rather than following some sort of physical stress. James B. Pierce, Ph.D., believes he has identified the cause of Prinzmetal's, which occurs most commonly at two specific times in the day, early morning and late afternoon, when magnesium levels are at their lowest.[40] Dr. Pierce estimates that up to 50 percent of sudden heart attacks may be due to magnesium deficiency. He found that magnesium worked better than nitroglycerine for his own stress-induced chest pains. In fact, Dr. Pierce could predict that he would get chest pain after a stressful day, a long drive, or an emotional upset and would increase his intake of magnesium to forestall symptoms.

Risk factors for angina include magnesium deficiency, smoking, diabetes mellitus, hyperlipidemia, type A personality, sedentary lifestyle, poor diet, and family history of coronary artery disease. Diagnosis of angina, to differentiate it from myocardial infarction and unstable angina, includes an EKG (electrocardiogram) taken during an angina attack; an exercise tolerance test, which is an EKG taken while on a treadmill; and a coronary angiogram (an X-ray view of dye in the coronary arteries) to assess whether the coronary arteries are open or blocked.

Once angina is diagnosed, the recommendations are universal: stop smoking, lose weight, get blood pressure under control (with or without drugs), and in extreme cases of arterial blockages, undergo bypass surgery to remove blocked arteries. The best treatment for angina, however, is prevention. By eliminating sugar, alcohol, and junk foods from your diet you help prevent heart disease, because these foods have no magnesium and serve only to create magnesium deficiency. When you eat a more balanced, non-processed-food diet, you have a better chance of increasing your magnesium intake. With magnesium and other heart-healthy supplements, a healthy diet and exercise regimen, you have a fighting chance of avoiding this epidemic. See page 108 for a list of supplements to cover all aspects of heart disease.

HEART ATTACKS

Myocardial infarction (MI), or heart attack, causes permanent damage to the heart muscle and requires immediate hospitalization. MI is the result of coronary artery disease due to atherosclerosis or due to spasms caused by magnesium deficiency. The artery may be damaged gradually by plaque, suddenly go into spasm, become blocked by a blood clot, or a combination of the above, often accelerated by excessive emotion. The calcified atherosclerotic plaque, the arterial spasm, and even the blood clot are all caused or worsened by magnesium deficiency.

Laboratory findings distinguish a heart attack from an episode of angina on the basis of heart muscle damage and certain heart enzyme levels that become elevated several hours after a heart attack and remain elevated for several days. The immediate treatment for an acute heart attack usually includes anticoagulant drugs in an intravenous drip. Intravenous magnesium given as soon as possible after a heart attack, however, may provide the best protection for the heart. Oral magnesium treatment also inhibits blood clots in patients with coronary artery disease whether the patient is on aspirin therapy or not.[41] As more doctors read the considerable research on magnesium they are incorporating magnesium into their intravenous and oral protocols for heart patients.

Magnesium has been studied for its effects on the heart

since the 1930s and used by injection for the treatment of heart conditions since the 1940s.[42,43] Magnesium's life-saving effects have been confirmed and reconfirmed in many clinics and laboratories. For example, in an analysis of seven major clinical studies, researchers concluded that magnesium (in doses of 5–10 g by intravenous injection) reduced the odds of death by an astounding 55 percent in acute MI.[44,45] Over the past decade, several large clinical trials using magnesium have shown its beneficial effects: If intravenous magnesium is given (1) before any other drugs and (2) immediately after onset of a heart attack, the incidence of high blood pressure, congestive heart failure, arrhythmia, or a subsequent heart attack is vastly reduced. One such study, called LIMIT-2, provided powerful evidence that early magnesium administration protects the heart muscle, prevents arrhythmia, and improves long-term survival.[46,47,48] Magnesium might improve the aftermath of acute heart attack by preventing rhythm problems; improving blood flow to the heart by dilating blood vessels; protecting the damaged heart muscle against calcium overload; improving heart muscle function; breaking down any blood clots blocking the arteries; and reducing free-radical damage. Magnesium may also help the heart drug digoxin to be more effective in the treatment of cardiac arrhythmia;[49] without enough magnesium, digoxin can become toxic.[50]

The suggested criteria for magnesium intervention were

not followed in a very large trial called ISIS-4, and the outcome did not show the same results as the LIMIT trial.[51] In the ISIS trial, magnesium was given many hours *after* the onset of symptoms and after blood clotting had begun. The two trials were as dissimilar as apples and oranges, yet the debate over magnesium's efficacy still rages. Since the LIMIT and ISIS studies, several smaller trials have shown even greater recovery from heart attacks using intravenous magnesium, including a trial of two hundred people with a 74 percent lower death rate.[52]

Pharmaceutical companies, who want to promote their own drug therapies, cite the ISIS trial as proof that magnesium sulfate doesn't work; supporters of magnesium cite the LIMIT trial as proof that it does. Your doctor may even be influenced by the ISIS trial and think magnesium is not an important option in your care. But cardiologists who are looking for alternatives to drug therapy and to its many side effects, and who read studies thoroughly, are using it. To help you find these doctors, there is a list in the Appendix of complementary medicine associations whose doctors study alternatives to the drug-based medicine they learned in medical school. Because one of the major side effects of heart medications, especially diuretics, is magnesium deficiency, it is vital that magnesium be tested with an ionized magnesium test and supplemented in heart patients who are on medication. The dosage ranges from 6 to 10 mg/kg/day (300–1,000 mg per day), but this should be taken only under a doctor's supervision if you are on any other heart medications. See page 108 for magnesium dosage.

SPASTIC HEART

Between 40 and 60 percent of people who suffer sudden heart attacks may actually have no arterial blockage or history of irregular heartbeats.[53] Two suspected causes are spasms in the coronary arteries and the occurrence of a severe heart rhythm disturbance, such as atrial fibrillation. Both of these conditions can be caused by a deficiency of magnesium. Low magnesium makes the heart muscle hyperirritable, leading to the development of a rhythm disturbance that can't be stopped without emergency medical intervention. An astute physician recognizes the possibility of magnesium deficiency and immediately gives magnesium intravenously, as in the LIMIT trial. Rapid heartbeat or atrial tachycardia, premature beats, and atrial fibrillation have all responded to treatment with IV magnesium.[54,55,56]

The most common time for the onset of heart attacks is around 9 A.M. on Mondays as people gird themselves for another long workweek.[57] As mentioned earlier, people who suffer from spasm-induced angina attacks most often experience them at the same time each day, usually in the morning and late afternoon, when magnesium levels are at their lowest. The morning deficiency is likely the result of overnight fasting and the loss of magnesium through the urine. Deficiency in the afternoon may be caused by depletion of magnesium induced by the stress of the day and not yet replenished by the evening meal. In view of this, it seems reasonable that people with angina, heart spasms, hypertension, or heart disease should consult with their doctors, take an ionized magnesium test, and, if it shows a deficiency, take at least 200 mg of magnesium three times each day; before breakfast, at 2 P.M., and before going to bed.

ARRHYTHMIA

Magnesium's ability to neutralize the heart-damaging effects of catecholamines (the products of stress-induced adrenaline and cortisol) is the miracle that can prevent many of the side effects of acute heart attack such as arrhythmia.[58] Magnesium deficiency contributes to abnormal heart rhythms, possibly because magnesium is responsible for maintaining normal potassium and sodium concentrations inside heart muscle cells. A balance of potassium, sodium, calcium, and magnesium allows for normal heart muscle contraction and maintains normal heartbeat. A central pacemaker within the heart muscle creates a normal pumping action that travels across the heart; cardiac arrhythmia occurs when other, less suitable areas of the heart are forced to assume the role of the central pacemaker when it becomes damaged or irritated by lack of oxygen due to blocked blood vessels, caused by drugs (including coffee), hormonal imbalance, or deficiency of magnesium. These new pacemakers are even more sensitive to magnesium deficiency and are responsive to magnesium therapy that has been successfully used for over sixty years.[59] Magnesium is also an accepted treatment for ventricular arrhythmias,[60,61] congestive heart failure where the heart is weak and unable to empty after each heartbeat,[62,63] and before and after heart surgery, including coronary bypass grafting.[64,65,66] All these studies indicate that the frequency of ventricular arrhythmias is reduced by administration of intravenous magnesium and support an early high-dose administration of intravenous magnesium in the wake of myocardial infarction.

MITRAL VALVE PROLAPSE

Magnesium deficiency has been implicated in mitral valve prolapse (MVP), a disorder in which the mitral valve fails to completely close off one of the heart chambers during heart contraction. It is also called floppy valve syndrome. Blood rushing through the open valve can be heard as a heart murmur with a stethoscope. When cardiac ultrasound became more commonplace, the diagnosis of MVP escalated, especially in young women. There is no allopathic treatment for the condition, and in mild and even moderate cases it doesn't cause any symptoms. However, patients are usually warned that they should take antibiotics when having dental work done to prevent the possibility of bacteria from the gums being picked up in the bloodstream and lodging on the prolapsed valve, causing infection. This is a very rare occurrence and some doctors disapprove of this overuse of antibiotics, but it remains a potential liability threat to dentists who don't warn their patients.

Dr. Melvyn Werbach, author of *Nutritional Influences on Disease*, believes that MVP is overdiagnosed and also maintains that it is a magnesium deficiency disease that is well treated by magnesium. The valves of the heart are pulled tight by muscles, which, like any other muscle in the body, depend on magnesium for proper functioning. The mitral valve prolapses because it is not held tight. Mildred Seelig reports that low magnesium levels have been found in as many as 85 percent of MVP patients.[67] Sixty percent of 141 individuals with strongly symptomatic MVP had low magnesium levels, compared to only 5 percent of the control group. Magnesium supplementation given for five weeks reduced the symptoms of chest pain, palpitation, anxiety, low energy, faintness, and difficulty breathing by about 50 percent.[68]

CHELATION THERAPY

Even alternative medicine can make more use of magnesium. Chelation therapy is an intravenous treatment with a chemical called EDTA that pulls out excess calcium and iron from the body to treat atherosclerosis and heart disease. It would be much more convenient to use magnesium as part of an oral chelation protocol preventively, to keep calcium from building up in the first place. When intravenous EDTA is used, however, generous amounts of magnesium are given as well.

SUPPLEMENTS FOR HEART DISEASE

Magnesium: 300 mg twice per day

Coenzyme Q_{10}: 30 mg three times a day

Bromelain: 500 mg three times a day between meals

Vitamin E as mixed tocopherols: 400 IU twice a day

Crategus tincture: 20 drops two to three times a day

Bioflavonoids rutin or quercetin: 500 mg daily

Biotin: 5 mg daily.

FOR ATHEROSCLEROSIS ADD:

Niacin (vitamin B_3): 100 mg three times a day, working up to 6 g daily. Do not use time-release niacin, which has been associated with liver damage. Niacinamide (which does not cause flushing) is not effective for lowering cholesterol.

Folic acid: 800 mcg daily

Vitamin B_6: 50 mg daily

Vitamin B complex: 50 mg per day

Vitamin C: 1,000 mg three times a day

Calcium: 1,000 mg daily (especially aids hypertension)

DIET FOR HEART DISEASE

A good diet is based on chicken, fish, whole grains, legumes, fruit, and vegetables. Therapeutic foods high in magnesium should be included: garlic, onions, nuts, seeds, wheat germ, and sprouts. Don't fall into the trap of blaming cholesterol above all else. Using margarine is not the answer to heart disease. The proper dietary fats for human consumption are butter, olive oil, flaxseed oil, and coconut oil. The diet for all forms of heart disease should exclude alcohol, coffee, white sugar, white flour, fried foods, and trans fatty acids (found in margarine, baked, fried, and processed foods).

CHAPTER 6

Syndrome X, Diabetes, and Sugar Imbalance

SYNDROME X

The term "syndrome X" describes a set of conditions that many believe is just another fancy name for the consequences of long-standing nutritional deficiency, especially magnesium deficiency. The long list includes hypertension, obesity, high cholesterol, elevated triglycerides, and elevated uric acid. This complex collectively appears to be caused by disturbed insulin metabolism (initiated by magnesium deficiency), called insulin resistance, and eventually leads to diabetes, angina, and heart attack. Syndrome X, according to Dr. Gerald Reaven, who coined the term, may be responsible for a large percentage of the heart and artery disease that occurs today. Unquestionably, magnesium deficiency is a major factor in the origins of each of its signs and symptoms, from elevated triglycerides and obesity to disturbed insulin metabolism.[1,2]

INSULIN RESISTANCE

Insulin's job is to open up sites on cell membranes to allow the influx of glucose, a cell's source of fuel. Cells that no longer respond to the advances of insulin and refuse the entry of glucose are called insulin-resistant. As a result, blood glucose levels rise and the body produces more and more insulin, to no avail. Glucose and insulin rampage throughout the body, causing tissue damage that results in magnesium deficiency, an increased risk of heart disease, and adult-onset diabetes. One of the major reasons the cells don't respond to insulin is lack of magnesium.[3] Some studies show that chronic insulin resistance in patients with adult-onset diabetes is associated with a reduction of magnesium; magnesium is necessary to allow glucose to enter cells.[4] Additional studies confirm that when insulin is released from the pancreas, magnesium in the cell normally responds and opens the cell to allow entry of glucose, but in the case of magnesium deficiency combined with insulin resistance the normal mechanisms just don't work.[5] Fortunately, the higher the levels of magnesium in the body, the greater the sensitivity of the cells to insulin and the possibility of reversing the problem.[6]

CARDIOVASCULAR METABOLIC SYNDROME (CVMS)

Dr. Larry Resnick of Cornell University, involved in heart and magnesium research for over twenty years, has another name for syndrome X, cardiovascular metabolic syndrome (CVMS), and he is closer to the truth when he says it is characterized by a high calcium-to-magnesium ratio. (Remember, too much calcium automatically creates a magnesium deficiency).[7] Americans in general have a high calcium-to-magnesium ratio in their diet and consequently in their bodies. Finland, which has the highest incidence of heart attack in middle-aged men in the world, also has a high calcium-to-magnesium ratio in the diet. The U.S. ratio in this study is said to be 3.5:1, Finland's 4:1.[8] (With our dietary emphasis on a high calcium intake without sufficient magnesium, according to magnesium expert Dr. Mildred Seelig, we will soon have a 6:1 ratio.) Although the recommended dietary ratio of calcium to magnesium is 2:1, in order to offset the deficiency that many people with syndrome X already have, it may be necessary to ingest one part calcium to one part magnesium in supplement form.

MAGNESIUM DEFICIENCY AND SYNDROME X

According to Dr. Resnick, syndrome X is caused not by chronically elevated insulin levels but by a low level of magnesium ions—because insufficient magnesium is the cause of insulin resistance in the first place.[9] As stated, insulin opens the cells to glucose only if the cells have sufficient amounts of magnesium, and without magnesium, insulin resistance occurs. Studies clearly show that animals deprived of dietary magnesium develop insulin resistance, and the human population has the same risk.[10] Some researchers conclude that hypertension and insulin resistance may just be different expressions of deficient levels of cellular magnesium.[11] The various conditions that make up syndrome X or CVMS all have similar magnesium-deficient origins.

The magnesium deficiency in syndrome X comes from a combination of our magnesium-deficient diets and the well-documented loss of magnesium in the urine caused by elevated insulin. A vicious cycle creates further magnesium losses, causing more syndrome X symptoms. The cornerstone of both prevention and treatment of syndrome X, along with diet, is to restore magnesium to normal levels. Unfortunately, for many, the ravages of diabetes, hypertension, and high cholesterol have taken their toll, but even then, magnesium taken along with medications can play a beneficial role in controlling and reducing symptoms.[12,13]

DIABETES

Diabetes is the seventh-leading cause of death in this country. There are sixteen million diabetics in the United States, with the numbers increasing dramatically as the population gets older and as more younger people succumb to a high-sugar diet. There are two main types of diabetes. About 10 percent of diabetics are labeled type I and are dependent on insulin. Type I diabetes usually develops in children; they may have suffered a viral infection of the pancreas, resulting in impaired or absent insulin production, and require insulin injections to replace their loss. Type II or

**THREE THINGS YOU NEED TO KNOW
ABOUT MAGNESIUM AND DIABETES**

1. Magnesium deficiency may be an independent predictor of diabetes.
2. Diabetics both need more magnesium and lose more than most people.
3. Magnesium is necessary for the production, function, and transport of insulin.

adult-onset diabetics tend to be non-insulin-dependent, overweight, and between fifty and seventy years old at onset. In type II diabetes, insulin is readily available but the cells of the body appear to be resistant to it. Insulin is unable to do its job of opening up the cell membrane to allow the passage of glucose into the cell to feed the furnace.

A third type of diabetes, gestational diabetes, is usually short-lived. This glucose intolerance may have been present but undetected before pregnancy but usually develops due to the stresses of pregnancy. Ionic magnesium testing demonstrates the presence of magnesium depletion in pregnancy itself and to a greater extent in gestational diabetes. Magnesium depletion, or relative calcium excess, may predispose women to vascular complications of pregnancy and needs to be addressed.[14] The ionic magnesium test is vitally important in diagnosing magnesium deficiency in gestational diabetes. Intervention with magnesium supplements can greatly improve the outcome for both mother and baby.

The signs and symptoms of diabetes are polydipsia (excessive thirst), polyuria (excessive urination), and polyphagia (excessive eating). In type I, weight loss may be the first sign, but type II diabetics are usually overweight. A common side effect of excessive sugar, which can be excreted through the urine and sweat, is an overgrowth of the yeast organism *Candida albicans*, resulting in rashes on the skin, especially under the breasts and in the groin, yeast vaginitis in women, and yeast discharge in men.

Common complications of diabetes include nerve damage, which mostly affects the feet, with symptoms of numbness, tingling, burning, and pain; atherosclerosis and heart attacks; damage to small blood vessels in the eyes and kidneys, causing vision loss (diabetes is the leading cause of blindness in the United States) and kidney disease; and diabetic foot ulcers, with increased susceptibility to infection, gangrene, and amputation. All these complications relate to magnesium deficiency and demonstrate the need for sensitive magnesium testing and magnesium supplementation for diabetes.[15]

Low magnesium, widely recognized as a marker for diabetes, occurs in up to 40 percent of diabetic patients.[16,17,18] Lack of magnesium increases the risk of cardiovascular disease, eye symptoms, and nerve damage in diabetics, whereas supplementation can prevent them.[19,20,21] Most importantly for diabetics, magnesium is a necessary cofactor in the production of energy from sugar stores in the muscles and liver.

Studies show that even moderate improvement of blood sugar control in patients with type I diabetes seems to reduce the loss of magnesium, increases serum HDL cholesterol (the good kind), and decreases serum triglycerides. These reductions in magnesium loss and serum triglycerides and the elevation of good cholesterol may reduce the risk of developing cardiovascular disease in patients with type I diabetes.[22]

HOW DID WE BECOME A NATION OF DIABETICS?

In non-Western cultures, it takes only one generation of people eating a diet high in refined sugar and flour to develop diabetes. This is true of people around the world, from Inuit to secluded African tribes. The immediate advice given to a newly diagnosed diabetic is to stop eating sugar and other refined carbohydrates. It is only common sense that avoiding these unhealthy nonfoods in the first place could greatly reduce the incidence of diabetes, yet the medical community has been slow to promote this idea.

Partly as a result, both obesity and adult-onset diabetes are on the rise in children. In the last decade, soft drink consumption has almost doubled among kids, adding an average of 15 to 20 extra teaspoons of sugar a day just from soda and other sugared drinks. These all-too-popular beverages account for more than a quarter of all drinks consumed in

LABORATORY FINDINGS IN DIABETES

- Blood glucose greater than or equal to 200 mg/dl (11.1 μmol/dl) two hours after an oral dose of 75 g of glucose dissolved in water
- Incidental blood glucose greater than or equal to 200 mg/dl (11.1 μmol/dl) in someone with signs and symptoms of diabetes
- High cholesterol
- Low magnesium ions

the United States. More than 15 billion gallons were sold in 2000.[23] A 2001 report in the prestigious medical journal *The Lancet* revealed that each additional soft drink a day gives a child a 60 percent greater chance of becoming obese.[24] Dr. France Bellisle, of France's Institute of Health and Medical Research, said the study provided convincing new evidence about the relationship between sugar and weight gain in children. It is unfortunate that it has taken so long for the *first* study on sugar and weight gain to be funded and published—so many children and adults are already addicted to sugar, and there is no turning back. Not until diabetes strikes does any medical body recommend cutting back on sugar intake.

We know from other important research that obese

children develop insulin resistance, a precursor to diabetes, fifty-three times more frequently than normal kids. The number of obese children in the United States doubled between 1980 and 1994; today 24 percent of kids are obese. Recently there has been a 70 percent rise in diabetes in thirty-year-olds, and the trend shows no sign of abating.

As a nation, we eat 140 pounds of sugar per year per person, so it is no wonder that more and more people are developing symptoms of diabetes and insulin resistance and suffering from magnesium deficiency. Even more shocking are studies on both animals and healthy adults that demonstrate a greatly depressed immune response to infection that lasts over five hours after the ingestion of 20 tsp of sugar.[25,26,27] Part of the danger with sugar is that you may not even realize how much you are ingesting. On ingredient labels, sugar is listed under carbohydrates and is often not distinguished from complex carbohydrates. Furthermore, the measurements are given in grams, even though most Americans think in teaspoons. People are stunned when I tell them there are 8 to 10 tsp of sugar in an ordinary soda (1 tsp of sugar is equivalent to 4.2 g).

Sugar overload can cause magnesium deficiency in several ways. Processed sugar is devoid of vitamins and minerals, leaving empty calories that provide no valuable nutrients. Nutritional research reported by Dr. Abram Hoffer (the originator, with Linus Pauling, of orthomolecular medicine) shows that the refining process of sugar removes 93 percent of chromium, 89 percent of manganese, 98 percent of cobalt, 83 percent of copper, 98 percent of zinc, and 98 percent of magnesium—all essential to life. In addition, the body has to tap into its own reserves of minerals and vitamins to ensure sugar's digestion.

Inability to utilize sugar results in the formation of toxic products such as pyruvic acid and other abnormal sugars that accumulate in the brain, nervous system, and red blood cells, where they interfere with cell respiration and hasten degenerative disease. Adding sugar to the diet produces an excessively acid condition in the body; to neutralize it the body has to draw upon its stores of the alkaline minerals calcium, magnesium, and potassium. If the acidic condition is severe, calcium and magnesium will even be taken from the bones and teeth, which leads to decay, softening, and ultimately osteoporosis.

In summary, magnesium plays a pivotal role in the secretion and function of insulin; without it, diabetes is inevitable. Measurable magnesium deficiency is common in diabetes and in many of its complications, including heart disease, eye damage, high blood pressure, and obesity. When the treatment of diabetes includes magnesium, these problems are prevented or minimized.[28] And we do know that magnesium-rich water in certain communities confers a protective effect against the disease.[29,30] Magnesium supplementation improves insulin response, improves glucose tolerance, and reduces the stickiness of red blood cell membranes.

Magnesium seems to be essential in the treatment of peripheral vascular disease associated with diabetes.[31] With long-term damage, however, many symptoms may be irreversible, even with adequate magnesium and associated nutrients.

DIET FOR DIABETES

The proper diet for the prevention and treatment of diabetes includes frequent small meals of protein (fish, chicken, and meat) and complex carbohydrates (whole grains, legumes, and vegetables) and the avoidance of simple sugars and white flour. Stevia, from the leaves of a plant that grows in South America, is the best sweetener to use. You can find it in health food stores. Don't use the sugar substitute aspartame, which, in certain individuals, has been shown to worsen blood sugar control and cause weight gain, headaches, nerve damage, and eye damage, because it is made partly from wood alcohol, which breaks down to formaldehyde.[32] Fiber from oat bran, flaxseed, and apples has a positive effect on keeping blood sugar balanced.

Alternative medicine practitioners also suggest identifying any existing food allergies by eliminating likely suspects (dairy, wheat, corn) from the diet for several days and then eating several meals of one of the suspected foods in one day and doing a blood test or finger stick for glucose. If the blood sugar is elevated after eating a particular food, it may be wise to avoid that food and find replacements that do not elevate the blood sugar.

SUPPLEMENTS FOR DIABETES

Magnesium: 300 mg twice per day

Vitamin E as mixed tocopherols: 400 IU twice a day

Bioflavonoids rutin or quercetin: 500 mg daily

Folic acid: 800 mcg daily

Vitamin B$_6$: 50 mg daily

Vitamin B complex: 50 mg per day

Vitamin C: 1,000 mg three times a day

Calcium: 1,000 mg daily

Chromium: chromium picolinate, 200–400 mcg daily, alternating with Brewer's yeast: 1 tbsp three times a day (contains glucose tolerance factor [GTF], which balances blood sugar) or specialized chromium (GTF): 200 mcg per day

Zinc picolinate: 15 mg daily

Copper: 2–4 mg daily

Selenium: 200 mcg daily

Manganese: 5 mg daily

Vanadium: 15 mg daily

Omega-3 fatty acids: 5 g daily

Garlic: one or two cloves daily

CHAPTER 7

PMS, Dysmenorrhea, Infertility, Polycystic Ovarian Syndrome, Preeclampsia, and Cerebral Palsy

THREE THINGS YOU NEED TO KNOW ABOUT MAGNESIUM AND PMS

1. Chocolate, which some women have a craving for when they're premenstrual, contains lots of magnesium, but the added sugar and fat make it far less desirable as a food.
2. The patent for Prozac has run out, so it has been patented under a new name, Sarafem, for PMS. PMS is not a Sarafem deficiency, but magnesium deficiency can cause some forms of PMS.
3. Magnesium is a safe treatment for PMS and PMS headaches.

Maureen didn't know what came over her every month, but she would get anxious and irritable and go on a chocolate binge. She tried to keep it to herself, but lately the other women at work had begun to make not-so-subtle comments and tease her about her "evil twin." Then Anna sat with her over lunch one day and told her about a support group she was leading for women with premenstrual syndrome. One of their self-help methods was to keep a journal of symptoms and to keep a food diary to see if eating certain foods coincided with having those symptoms.

Maureen's journal for the next couple of months clearly showed that her symptoms of anxiety, fluid retention, sugar and chocolate cravings, mood swings, irritability, bloating, edema, headache, and sore breasts escalated before her period and lifted the minute her period began.

Taking magnesium supplements may be the solution, advises Melvyn Werbach, M.D. Recent studies showed that of 192 women taking 400 mg of magnesium daily for PMS, 95 percent experienced less breast pain and had less weight gain, 89 percent suffered less nervous tension, and 43 percent had fewer headaches. (Dr. Werbach and several other researchers also advise that women should take 50 mg of vitamin B_6 daily with the magnesium to assist in magnesium absorption.)[1] Red blood cell magnesium tests show low levels of magnesium in women with PMS.[2] Even total serum magnesium levels, which are low only when there is a severe magnesium deficiency, diminished significantly in the premenstrual week in a group of forty women.[3] In a small trial of thirty-two women, oral magnesium was found to be an effective treatment of premenstrual symptoms related to mood changes.[4] Treatment with magnesium eases headaches, sugar cravings, low blood sugar, and dizziness related to PMS.[5,6]

In another innovative research study, magnesium ion levels were taken at several times during normal menstrual cycles to determine magnesium and calcium levels in relation to menstrual phases.[7] There was a comparatively high magnesium ion level in the first week after the onset of the period, a statistically significant decrease in magnesium ions around the time of ovulation, and a large decrease in magnesium ions and total serum magnesium when the serum progesterone concentration peaked in the third week. There was also a significant increase in the serum-calcium-to-magnesium ratio at both the time of ovulation and the fourth week after the onset of the period. That calcium-to-magnesium imbalance can cause premenstrual symptoms during the last week of the menstrual cycle. The good news is that you can take care of it easily by taking the right amounts of calcium and magnesium. For most women this translates into equal amounts of calcium and magnesium, 600–1,000 mg of each a day in divided doses.

An elegant new study demonstrates that estrogen and progesterone, the female sex hormones, influence magnesium ion levels in the body, which may help explain why magnesium relieves symptoms of PMS, including migraine, bloating, and edema.[8] Exposure of cultured smooth muscle cells from brain blood vessels to a low concentration of estrogen did not interfere with the level of magnesium ions. However, exposure to increased concentrations of estrogen induced significant loss of magnesium ions; at the highest concentration, the level of magnesium ions decreased approximately 30 percent in comparison with controls. Exposure of the cultured cells to a low concentration of progesterone resulted in an increased level of magnesium ions. However, when these cells were exposed to higher concentrations of progesterone, cellular levels of magnesium ions decreased significantly. The higher the estrogen or progesterone concentration, the lower the levels of magnesium ions.

The data in this experiment indicate that the normally low concentrations of the female sex hormones, estrogen and progesterone, help cerebral vascular smooth muscle cells sustain normal concentrations of magnesium ions, which are beneficial to vascular function, whereas high levels of estrogen and progesterone significantly deplete magnesium ions, possibly resulting in cerebral vessel spasms and reduced cerebral blood flows—and thus leading to premenstrual syndrome and migraine and possible stroke risk. These findings help to explain why more women than men suffer migraines, and why migraines occur more frequently in the second half of the menstrual cycle, when estrogen and progesterone are both elevated.

Guy Abraham, M.D., a retired obstetrician and gynecologist, is a widely published author who has pursued major research on premenstrual syndrome. Dr. Abraham identifies four types of PMS, each of which has distinct characteristics related to hormonal fluctuations.

1. PMS-A (anxiety), with symptoms of mood swings, nervous tension, irritability, anxiety. Related to high estrogen, low progesterone.
2. PMS-C (craving), with symptoms of increased appetite, headache, fatigue, dizziness, fainting, palpitations. Related to increased carbohydrate intake and decreased prostaglandin E1–type foods (from fish, nuts, seeds).
3. PMS-D (depression), with symptoms of depression, crying, forgetfulness, confusion, insomnia. Related to low estrogen, high progesterone, elevated male hormone with excess hair growth.
4. PMS-H (hyperhydration), with symptoms of fluid retention, weight gain, swollen extremities, breast tenderness, abdominal bloating. Related to excess aldosterone (a kidney hormone that causes fluid retention).

Maureen had symptoms from three of the four groups. Her successful treatment involved balancing hormones and replacing deficient nutrients. She began to take a daily tablespoon of flax oil, which contains omega-3 essential fatty acids, along with magnesium, vitamin B$_6$, and calcium. Essential fatty acids are necessary building blocks for hormone production as long as they have magnesium and B vitamins as cofactors.

PMS AND YOUR DIET

A fascinating diet review shows that women suffering from PMS followed diets that were

275 percent higher in refined sugar
79 percent higher in dairy products
78 percent higher in sodium
77 percent lower in magnesium
63 percent higher in refined carbohydrates
53 percent lower in iron
52 percent lower in zinc[9]

Ounce for ounce, chocolate has more magnesium than any other food, and the irresistible urge to consume chocolate is a sure sign of magnesium deficiency. Premenstrual chocolate craving is widespread because magnesium is at its lowest around that time of a woman's menses. The answer is not to eat more chocolate, however, but to increase magnesium intake by eating more nuts, whole grains, seafood, and green vegetables, and by taking magnesium supplements. The chocolate cravings will vanish when there is enough magnesium in the diet.

Other foods to consume in moderation are beef and chicken, which are frequently treated with synthetic

---

PMS AND DEPRESSION

Women can get depressed before their period, but PMS is not just depression. Yet PMS is often considered by medical doctors and pharmaceutical companies to be a psychiatric condition suitable for treatment with selective serotonin reuptake inhibitors such as fluoxetine (Prozac, Sarafem). But remember that a lack of fluoxetine does not cause PMS symptoms; a lack of magnesium does. The replacement of magnesium in the body will treat PMS and cause no side effects. In fact, it has also been found that magnesium relieves the depression of premenstrual syndrome by positively influencing serotonin activity naturally. Sarafem has no such claim.

---

hormones. Remember that one type of PMS occurs when there is too much estrogen and too little progesterone in a woman's body. It is possible to end up with too much estrogen stimulation by eating, drinking, or breathing hormones, pesticides, or other chemical residues that mimic estrogen. The saturated fat and arachidonic acid in meat also suppress progesterone production and cause symptoms of inflammation that worsen PMS and can lead to painful periods. Essential fatty acids from fish, nuts, and seeds, including flaxseed, are much healthier fats and help prevent PMS, unless you have a magnesium deficiency. Without magnesium, essential fatty

TREATMENT FOR PMS

DIET

Increase complex carbohydrates and fiber.

Reduce saturated fats, particularly red meat and dairy.

Eliminate caffeine and alcohol.

Reduce salt intake.

Eliminate sugar.

SUPPLEMENTS

Magnesium: 300–600 mg daily

Vitamin B_6: 100 mg three times a day for ten days before the period starts

Vitamin B complex: 50 mg daily

Vitamin E as mixed tocopherols: 400 IU daily

Essential fatty acids: flaxseed oil, 1 tbsp twice per day, or evening primrose oil, 500 mg three times per day

Calcium: 1,000 mg daily

Progesterone: ¼ tsp twice a day rubbed into the skin (rotate inner thighs, stomach, inner arms). Use natural progesterone cream derived from wild yam to balance excess estrogen. It should contain USP progesterone 450–500 mg/oz (have a naturopathic doctor evaluate your hormones by testing levels in your saliva).

Milk thistle: 250 mg three times a day, to detox the liver

acids are not processed properly and are not able to calm the irritability and inflammation of PMS and painful periods. Magnesium deficiency is created by stress, which is common to PMS sufferers. The only solution to this vicious circle is to eat a healthy diet—organic, if possible—and take nutrient supplements that include magnesium.

DYSMENORRHEA (PAINFUL PERIODS)

Calcium can act like a painkiller and relaxant, but it may create these effects by driving magnesium out of the cells and into the bloodstream, where it is able to be directed toward ailing tissues to treat pain. So taking calcium can alleviate menstrual cramps in this way, but taking magnesium *before* your period may forestall the pain. A series of European studies with small groups of women who suffered painful periods consistently showed relief of symptoms with high doses of magnesium.[10,11,12] A balanced calcium and magnesium supplement (500 mg calcium and 300 mg magnesium, twice per day) helps to ensure adequate levels of both minerals and should be taken preventively. Extra magnesium can also be taken when the pain is at its worst (300 mg once or twice a day).

Some women find that decreasing their intake of meat before their period helps prevent cramps. What may not be obvious is that when you cut back on meat you have a better chance of eating more magnesium-rich foods that will ease symptoms of painful periods.

INFERTILITY

Dr. Sherry Rogers, a diplomate in family practice, allergy-asthma-immunology, and environmental medicine and a fellow of the American College of Nutrition, says that just as migraines are cerebral spasms, spasms in the fallopian tubes cause infertility. This may explain why so many infertile women get pregnant when they go on a whole-foods diet and take supplements including magnesium.[13] Magnesium is required in higher amounts during pregnancy.[14] So taking it to enhance conception also creates a healthier pregnancy.

POLYCYSTIC OVARIAN SYNDROME

Polycystic ovarian syndrome (PCOS) patients have a high incidence of insulin resistance and glucose intolerance. In a recent consultation, a young woman told me she had been advised to go on diabetic drugs, not because she has diabetes but because she has PCOS and the drugs were supposed to lower her insulin resistance. PCOS patients also tend to be at risk for hypertension, diabetes, and heart disease. Since a low magnesium ion level and a high calcium/magnesium ratio are associated with insulin resistance, cardiovascular problems, diabetes mellitus, and hypertension, a study was done on a group of PCOS patients to determine the effects of magnesium intervention. Significantly lower levels of magnesium ions and total serum magnesium and a significantly higher calcium-ion-to-magnesium-ion ratio were found in the PCOS patients compared with the controls, which gave me enough evidence to recommend a magnesium supplement of 300 mg twice per day to treat my patient's insulin resistance and possibly her PCOS as well.[15]

SEIZURES IN THE DELIVERY SUITE

Marie was not having a good pregnancy. She had gained too much weight, she had headaches, and her ankles and hands were swollen with edema. She also felt a tightness in her head and shortness of breath. At her eight-month visit to the doctor, her blood pressure was elevated, she had hyperactive reflexes, and her urine showed protein and sugar, the symptoms of preeclampsia (also called pregnancy-induced hypertension or toxemia). Preeclampsia occurs in 7 percent of all pregnancies and, according to the Preeclampsia Foundation, is responsible for at least seventy-six thousand maternal deaths worldwide each year. A rapidly progressive condition characterized by high blood pressure, hyperactive reflexes, edema, headaches, changes in vision, and protein in the urine, it can escalate and cause seizures, at which point it is called eclampsia.

Eclampsia is a serious condition that can cause premature labor, premature birth, and cerebral palsy in the newborn. Marie's doctor said that bed rest was the only solution to lower her blood pressure but that if she continued to have high blood pressure around the time of delivery, he would give her intravenous magnesium. Unfortunately, he did not have her current magnesium levels tested. Many researchers and clinicians recommend that pregnant women have an ionized magnesium test and take 300–600 mg of supplemental magnesium.[16,17,18] (Always check with your obstetrician or health care provider before adding any supplement, but know that magnesium has proven to be safe for both mother and child.)

Although magnesium is the treatment of choice for pregnancy-induced hypertension, it could be used more

Magnesium sulfate given intravenously for eclampsia has been used successfully for more than seventy-five years.[19] In the 1960s, the advent of new diuretics and anticonvulsant drugs threatened to displace magnesium sulfate. Drug companies continue to run expensive clinical trials to compare their newest antihypertensives and anti-convulsants to magnesium sulfate. Most studies show that magnesium is, in fact, more effective than synthetic medications, decreases both infant and maternal mortality, and is extremely safe. As one researcher remarked, "The significant improvement in fetal outcome with dietary magnesium supports the concept of magnesium supplementation during pregnancy."[20]

widely. Many researchers suggest that pregnant mothers routinely take magnesium to prevent complications during delivery and postpartum, and to help prevent premature births.[21] Clinical trials have demonstrated that mothers supplementing with magnesium oxide have larger, healthier babies and lower rates of preeclampsia, premature labor, sudden infant death, and birth defects, including cerebral palsy.[22]

Fortunately, Marie consulted a midwife specializing in preeclampsia, who was familiar with the use of magnesium in pregnancy. They checked the label of Marie's prenatal supplement and found that it contained only 150 mg of magnesium; she really needed at least 360 mg just to meet the RDA (recommended daily allowance) for pregnant women. The midwife recommended that Marie take a magnesium supplement to give her a total of 400 mg of elemental magnesium per day and to increase her intake of magnesium-rich foods.

On this new regimen, Marie noticed many positive changes. She had less back and neck tension, was no longer constipated (a common side effect of pregnancy), had more energy, and lost a lot of her edema and puffiness. Finally, the tightness in her head lessened and her blood pressure began to go down. When she told all this to her obstetrician, he actually apologized for not being more aware of her magnesium status and said it was a good reminder for him to be more diligent about his patients' prenatal supplements.

SIDS

Magnesium deficiency has been implicated in sudden infant death syndrome (SIDS), which has features in common with sudden cardiac death (SCD) of adults[23] and may be prevented by giving adequate magnesium to the mother and child.[24] An episode of muscular weakness induced by magnesium deficiency could prevent a distressed infant from turning its head when lying facedown and thus result in suffocation.[25]

The triple-risk model for SIDS describes the intersection of three potential risks: (1) a vulnerable newborn who is magnesium-deficient, (2) a critical adjustment and development period in a newborn displaying hyperirritability and unsettled cardiovascular and respiratory control, and (3) an outside stressor such as high-pitched noise, excessive motion or handling, chill, fever, or vaccination. Together, these three risks may trigger a shocklike episode of apnea, unconsciousness, and slow heart rate. Researchers feel that it is likely that a high proportion of SIDS deaths could be prevented by simple oral magnesium supplementation to infants during the first critical weeks and months of life.[26]

Dr. Jean Durlach, a professor at St. Vincent de Paul Hospital in Paris and president of the International Society for the Development of Research on Magnesium (SDRM), states, "This simple and cheap supplementation with doses of 300 milligrams per day to the mother is ethically justifiable. Furthermore the beneficial effects of magnesium supplementation are well established for the mother, for fetal development, and for the baby at birth." He calls for a large clinical trial of magnesium supplementation in pregnant and breast-feeding women.[27]

CEREBRAL PALSY

Cerebral palsy (CP) can occur when there is a fetal brain hemorrhage during the last stages of pregnancy, either from the mother's high blood pressure or from a lack of oxygen to the developing baby's brain. It can also be caused by low birth weight and prematurity. In cerebral palsy, the brain is damaged and is unable to properly direct muscle function. The brain gives the muscles contradictory signals, and as a result, the muscles lock and become spastic or go limp, creating a disabling and incurable condition. Close to half the infants born with CP also have mental handicaps. Very low birth weight babies (less than 1,500 g, or 3.3 lbs) are a hundred times more likely to have disabling CP than infants of average birth weight (3,000–3,500 g); more than 25 percent of all CP occurs in very low birth weight babies. More than half a million Americans suffer from CP, with estimated medical costs of $5 billion a year.

Since there is no treatment for CP, preventing cerebral palsy would be "very desirable indeed," asserts neurologist Karin B. Nelson of the National Institutes of Health in Bethesda, Maryland. Dr. Nelson and her colleagues concluded a groundbreaking study in 1995 showing that very low birth weight babies in four centers in California had a lower incidence of cerebral palsy when their mothers were treated with magnesium sulfate shortly before birth.[28] "This intriguing finding means that use of a simple medication could significantly decrease the incidence of cerebral palsy and prevent lifelong disability and suffering for thousands of Americans," said Zach W. Hall, Ph.D., director of the National Institute of Neurological Disorders and Stroke. The researchers calculated that magnesium sulfate reduced the prevalence of cerebral palsy by about 90 percent and reduced the prevalence of mental retardation by about 70 percent. They speculate that magnesium may play a role in brain development and possibly prevent cerebral hemorrhage in preterm infants.

Dr. Diane Schendel found very similar results the following year while studying a population in Atlanta.[29] Those mothers receiving magnesium sulfate delivered infants with a 90 percent lower prevalence of cerebral palsy and a 70 percent lower prevalence of mental retardation. The researchers reported that at one year of age, only 1 out of 113 babies whose mothers received magnesium sulfate developed cerebral palsy. Only two of the babies had mental handicaps. In contrast, 30 of the 405 children whose mothers did not receive magnesium sulfate had cerebral palsy and 22 had handicaps. The investigators speculated that magnesium may prevent fetal brain hemorrhage or block the harmful effects of a diminished oxygen supply to the brain. And for those babies exposed to too much oxygen in an attempt to overcome intrauterine deficits, magnesium protects the lungs.[30] A recent literature review and new research suggest that magnesium chloride might be even more protective for the developing brain than magnesium sulfate.[31,32]

Beyond magnesium supplementation given to expectant mothers and to newborns, there are certain interventions that can prevent some of the subsequent brain damage to low birth weight infants. One is specialized cranial massage provided within hours or days of birth by licensed practitioners. Naturopaths can help identify food or airborne allergies that can worsen symptoms, and can recommend a wholesome diet and supplement program. Be warned that many supplements on the shelf contain aspartame, a potent neurotoxin. You should never expose your child to this chemical.

SUPPLEMENTS FOR CHILDREN
WITH CEREBRAL PALSY

Magnesium: 10 mg/kg/day

Zinc: 5 mg per day

Vitamin B complex: 10 mg per day

Vitamin C: 200 mg per day

Bioflavonoids: 100 mg per day

Essential fatty acids: DHA, 1 tsp per day; cod liver oil,
   1 tsp per day; flaxseed oil, 1 tsp per day

CHAPTER 8

Osteoporosis and Kidney Stones

THREE THINGS YOU NEED TO KNOW ABOUT MAGNESIUM, OSTEOPOROSIS, AND KIDNEY STONES

1. Magnesium is just as important as calcium to prevent and treat osteoporosis.
2. Magnesium keeps calcium dissolved in the blood so it will not form kidney stones.
3. Taking calcium without magnesium for osteoporosis can promote kidney stones.

Muriel wondered how she managed to have soft bones and kidney stones all at the same time. Her recent bone density test showed obvious osteoporosis, yet she was now in the hospital with her third kidney stone attack. A young intern explained that she was losing calcium from her bones, which was being deposited in her kidneys and flushed out as hard, jagged crystals that were excruciatingly painful to pass. The high doses of calcium that she was taking for her osteoporosis were only making matters worse.

Muriel's urologist did an analysis on her kidney stones and told her to stop eating all dairy products and to avoid calcium supplements, but Muriel was very concerned that her osteoporosis would worsen.

When she came to see me, I was able to explain that there are approximately eighteen nutrients essential for healthy bones, including magnesium, the most important mineral after calcium. Susan Brown, Ph.D., director of the Osteoporosis Education Project in Syracuse, New York, warns that "the use of calcium supplementation in the face of magnesium deficiency can lead to a deposition of calcium in the soft tissue such as the joints, promoting arthritis, or in the kidney, contributing to kidney stones."[1] Dr. Brown recommends a daily dose of 450 mg of magnesium for the prevention and treatment of osteoporosis.

Women with osteoporosis have lower-than-average levels of magnesium in their diets, according to survey reports. Magnesium deficiency can compromise calcium metabolism and also hinder the body's production of vitamin D, further weakening bones.

Magnesium's role in bone health is multifaceted.

- Adequate levels of magnesium are essential for the absorption and metabolism of calcium.
- Magnesium stimulates a particular hormone, calcitonin, that helps to preserve bone structure and draws calcium out of the blood and soft tissues back into the bones, preventing some forms of arthritis and kidney stones.
- Magnesium suppresses another bone hormone called parathyroid, preventing it from breaking down bone.
- Magnesium converts vitamin D into its active form so that it can help calcium absorption.
- Magnesium is also required to activate an enzyme that is necessary to form new bone.
- Magnesium regulates active calcium transport.

With all these roles for magnesium to play, it is no wonder that even a mild deficiency can be a risk factor for osteoporosis. Further, if there is too much calcium in the body, especially from calcium supplementation, as in Muriel's case, magnesium absorption can be greatly impaired, resulting in worsening osteoporosis and the likelihood of kidney stones, arthritis, and heart disease.

Other factors that are important in the development of osteoporosis include diet, drugs, endocrine imbalance, allergies, vitamin D deficiency, and lack of exercise. A detailed review of the osteoporosis literature shows that chronically low intake of magnesium, vitamin D, boron, and vitamins K, B_{12}, B_6, and folic acid lead to osteoporosis. Similarly, chronically high intake of protein, sodium chloride, alcohol, and caffeine adversely affect bone health.[2,3] The typical Western diet (high in protein, salt and refined, processed foods) combined with an increasing sedentary lifestyle contributes to the increasing incidence of osteoporosis.

Looking at her lifestyle, Muriel saw how much she had contributed to her own condition. She averaged five cups of coffee, three glasses of wine, and twenty cigarettes a day. This was causing calcium and magnesium, and the other nutrients that have to deal with toxins, to be overworked or flushed out of her body. Her diet was mostly nutrient-deficient fast food because she was constantly on the run. She drank a lot of soda, which is high in phosphorus and causes calcium and magnesium to be eliminated. She also avoided the sun and therefore got little vitamin D.

Instead of becoming discouraged, Muriel was able to look on the bright side. At least now she knew what lifestyle habits she had to change and what supplements to take. Her kidney stones soon became a thing of the past, her overall health dramatically improved, and after two years there was actually an increase in her bone density.

OSTEOPOROSIS MISUNDERSTOOD
AND MISTREATED

Osteoporosis is neither a normal nor inevitable consequence of aging: Our bones were designed to last a lifetime. Popular wisdom, however, is that osteoporosis in women is due to a decrease in estrogen levels with age. Doctors therefore rely on estrogen, calcium, and drugs that stimulate bone formation to treat osteoporosis. The National Institutes of Health (NIH) Osteoporosis Prevention, Diagnosis, and Therapy Consensus Statement of 2000 was developed from a conference including eighty experts, but no mention of magnesium deficiency as a causative factor in osteoporosis was made in the final report.[4] With drug companies funding most of the osteoporosis research, there are very few large clinical trials investigating the magnesium connection in bone production. Although I found over twenty-two thousand journal articles on osteoporosis, there were only ten in the past decade that studied the magnesium connection in humans. As long as people are given false hope that there is some magic bullet in the pharmaceutical pipeline that will "cure" osteoporosis, or any other chronic disease, they will ignore the underlying reasons for their health problems.

Nonetheless, when you read the literature, there is ample evidence that many nutrients, especially magnesium, play a large role in bone development. Much animal research, for example, proves that magnesium depletion alters bone and mineral metabolism, which results in bone loss and osteoporosis.[5,6] Magnesium deficiency is very common in women with osteoporosis compared to controls.[7]

In one study, postmenopausal women with osteoporosis were able to stop the progression of the disease with 250–750 mg of magnesium daily for two years. Without any other added measures, 8 percent of these women experienced a net increase in bone density.[8] A group of menopausal women given a magnesium hydroxide supplement for two years had fewer fractures and significant increase in bone density.[9] Another study showed that by taking magnesium lactate (1,500–3,000 mg daily for two years), 65 percent of the women were completely free of pain and had no further degeneration of spinal vertebrae.[10] Magnesium in conjunction with hormonal replacement improved bone density in several groups of women compared to controls.[11,12] In fact, if you are taking estrogen and have a low magnesium intake, calcium supplementation may increase your risk of thrombosis (blood clotting that can lead to a heart attack).[13]

It is unfortunate that the treatment for osteoporosis has been simplified into the single battle cry "Take calcium." Calcium dominates every discussion about osteoporosis, is used to fortify dozens of foods (including orange juice and cereal), and is a top-selling supplement, but it cannot stand alone. In Chapter 1, we talked about the dance of calcium and magnesium. These minerals work so closely together that the lack of one immediately diminishes the effectiveness of the other. Even though the use of calcium supplementation for the management of osteoporosis has increased significantly in the last decade, scientific studies do not support such large doses after menopause. Soft tissue calcification could be a serious side effect of taking too much calcium.[14]

Osteoporosis is generally a progressive disease, and some say it is incurable, but if you avoid the risk factors, take a good range of bone-building nutrients, and exercise, you can halt the condition even if you have the symptoms. Prevention is the best defense, the key elements of which are:

- Eat a balanced, nutrient-rich diet
- Take supplements of calcium, magnesium, and the various bone support factors
- Practice a vigorous exercise program throughout life

DIET FOR OSTEOPOROSIS

A high-protein diet, excess sugar, alcohol, and coffee all rob the body of essential minerals. Prevention in the form of fruit and vegetables containing large amounts of calcium, magnesium, and potassium contributes to maintenance of bone mineral density.[15] Add more vegetables, whole grains, legumes, nuts, and seeds to your diet, and be sure to include some of the magnesium-rich foods listed on pages 218–219. The foods that are high in calcium are usually abundant in magnesium as well, including nuts and seeds, sardines, bok choy (Chinese cabbage), and broccoli.

SUPPLEMENTS FOR OSTEOPOROSIS

Calcium: 800 mg per day (organic veal bone is the best source, followed by calcium lactate, calcium citrate, or calcium malate)

Magnesium: 300 mg twice a day

Boron: 2 mg daily (involved in vitamin D conversion)

Copper: 1–3 mg daily (for collagen cross-linking)

Manganese: 5–10 mg per day (stimulates the production of mucopolysaccharides, the organic matrix of bone)

Zinc: 10 mg daily (important for bone matrix)

Vitamin A: 20,000 IU daily (forms bone matrix)

Vitamin B_6: 50 mg per day

Folic acid: 5 mg daily

Vitamin B complex: 50 mg per day

Vitamin C: 1,000 mg per day

Vitamin D: 400 IU daily (for calcium absorption)

Progesterone for postmenopausal women under the advice of your doctor and after hormonal saliva testing to determine deficiency of progesterone: days 1–25, use ¼ tsp of progesterone cream, rubbed into the skin, twice a day; take a break days 25–31 (make sure the product contains USP progesterone)

You can obtain about half your mineral needs from good organic foods. The supplement doses on the previous page assume that you are already getting minerals in your diet. If you do not eat a good diet, your mineral supplement amounts should be increased by 50 percent.

KIDNEY STONES

Kidney stones occur when the microscopic debris excreted in the urine becomes too concentrated to pass freely out of the kidneys into the bladder. Kidney stones are quite common in the general population. Risk factors for kidney stones include a history of hypertension and a low dietary intake of magnesium.[16] One percent of autopsies reveal stones in the urinary tract, but most are small enough to pass unnoticed. Up to 15 percent of white men and 6 percent of all women will develop one stone, with recurrence in

Most kidney stones are made up of calcium phosphate, calcium oxalate, or uric acid. Calcium stones are seen chiefly in men, often with a family history. Calcium phosphate and calcium oxalate alone are responsible for almost 85 percent of all stones. Uric acid stones make up 5–10 percent of all stones. They are also seen mostly in men, half of whom have gout. The remaining 5 percent are rare stones that can be formed during kidney infections.

about half of these people. Approximately one in a thousand people in the United States is hospitalized annually with excruciatingly painful stones trapped in their urinary passages. The pain begins in the lower back and can radiate across the abdomen or into the genitals or the inside of the thigh.

Diagnosis is made by urinalysis and X ray. A few calcium crystals or small stones often need no treatment but may be relieved with painkillers and muscle relaxants. Larger stones are treated with surgery or with lithotripsy (the breakdown of the stones into little pieces using special ultrasound machines).

Several factors can be involved in stone formation:

1. Elevated calcium in the urine is caused by a diet high in sugar, fructose, alcohol, coffee, and meat. These acidic foods pull calcium from the bone and excrete it through the kidneys. Calcium supplementation also causes elevated calcium in the urine.

2. Higher-than-normal levels of oxalate found in the urine may relate to a high dietary intake of oxalic-acid-containing foods: rhubarb, spinach, raw parsley, chocolate, tea, and coffee. The oxalic acid in them promotes stone formation by binding to calcium, creating insoluble calcium oxalate.

3. Dehydration concentrates calcium and other minerals in the urine. Six to eight glasses of water a day are an essential requirement for flushing the kidneys

properly. Increased sweating and not enough water intake create concentrated urine.

4. Soft drinks containing phosphoric acid encourage kidney stones in some people by pulling calcium out of the bones and depositing it in the kidneys.

Kidney stones and magnesium deficiency share the same list of causes, including a diet high in sugar, alcohol, oxalates, and coffee. An important animal study shows that a high dietary intake of fructose (from high-fructose corn syrup, used as a sweetener) significantly increases kidney calcification, especially when dietary magnesium is low.[17] The U.S. Department of Agriculture warns that young people, especially, derive too many of their daily calories from the high-fructose corn syrup in sodas and eat few greens, which are rich in magnesium. The phosphoric acid in soft drinks is also punishing to the magnesium in the body and depletes magnesium stores while wearing away bone.[18,19]

One of magnesium's many jobs is to keep calcium in solution to prevent it from solidifying into crystals; even at times of dehydration, if there is sufficient magnesium, calcium will stay in solution. Magnesium is the pivotal treatment for kidney stones. If you don't have enough magnesium to help dissolve calcium, you will end up with various forms of calcification. This translates into stones, muscle spasms, fibrositis, fibromyalgia, and atherosclerosis (calcification of the arteries).

Dr. George Bunce has clinically proven the relationship between kidney stones and magnesium deficiency.[20] As early as 1964, Bunce reported the benefits of administering a 420 mg dose of magnesium oxide per day to patients with histories of frequent stone formation.

When there is more calcium than magnesium, kidney stones can form. Let's look at that simple experiment from Chapter 1 again to prove the point. Crush and stir a calcium tablet in 1 ounce of water; note how much dissolves and how much is still swirling around in the bottom of the glass. Then add a crushed magnesium tablet, or the contents from a magnesium capsule, to the water and see how much more calcium dissolves. If calcium is dissolved properly in the blood, then it won't form crystals in the kidney.

Several older studies show the benefits of magnesium hydroxide in preventing stone formation. Fifty-five patients with a combined 480 stones in the previous ten years were placed on 200 mg of magnesium hydroxide daily. Patients were followed for two to four years, and only eight patients developed new stones. Of a group of forty-three kidney stone patients who did not receive magnesium, 59 percent developed new kidney stones over a four-year period.[21] An even earlier study using magnesium oxide and vitamin B_6 (a natural diuretic) showed a decrease in stone formation for 149 patients, who went from an average of 1.3 stones per year to 0.1 stones. Patients were followed for between four and a half and six years.[22] In another study, fifty-six patients were given 200 mg of magnesium hydroxide twice per day. At the two-year mark, forty-five were free of kidney stone recurrence; of thirty-four patients not taking magnesium, fifteen had recurrences after two years.[23]

Other studies show that urinary magnesium concentration is abnormally low and urinary calcium concentration is abnormally high in more than 25 percent of patients with kidney stones. Supplemental magnesium intake corrects this abnormality and prevents the recurrence of stones. Other researchers acknowledge that magnesium oxide or magnesium hydroxide therapy causes a considerable lessening of kidney stone recurrence in men and feel that soft tissue calcifications can be stopped and even prevented by magnesium therapy.[24] Magnesium seems to be as effective against stone formation as diuretics, the major drug treatment for kidney stones.[25] Avoidance of calcium, taking diuretics, and mechanical intervention, however, seem to be the current medical approach to kidney stones.

Epidemiological findings round out the picture of kidney stone occurrence and its association with low magnesium intake. The disease pattern in Greenland includes a low incidence of heart disease and kidney and urinary tract stones, few cases of diabetes mellitus, and little osteoporosis, all of which may be related to low calcium and high magnesium in their diet.[26]

DIETARY TREATMENT FOR KIDNEY STONES

On a regular basis, drink six to eight glasses of water a day; increase intake of green vegetables and fiber (vegetarians have a 40–60 percent decreased risk of stone formation) and foods high in magnesium, such as seeds, vegetables, and whole grains; and decrease consumption of sugar, alcohol, coffee, and meat.

For uric acid kidney stones, decrease consumption of high-purine foods such as alcohol, anchovies, herring, lentils, meat, mushrooms, organ meats, sardines, seafood, meats, and shellfish. For oxalate stones, decrease consumption of foods high in oxalic acid: red beet tops, black tea, cocoa, cranberry, nuts, parsley, tomatoes, rhubarb, and spinach. The citric acid in lemons, limes, oranges, pineapples, and gooseberries dissolves calcium oxalate and calcium phosphate, preventing stone formation.

SUPPLEMENTS FOR KIDNEY STONES

Magnesium: 300 mg twice per day
Calcium: 800 mg daily
Vitamin B_6: 50–100 mg daily

PART THREE

The Research Continues

While research identifying magnesium deficiency as a causative factor in heart disease, migraines, and eclampsia is clear-cut, many investigators believe that magnesium also plays an important role in chronic fatigue syndrome, fibromyalgia, environmental illness, and aging. More investigation needs to be done on these conditions to prove that magnesium deficiency is a contributing factor and that magnesium replacement should be part of the treatment protocol. Let's review what many clinicians and researchers already know about these conditions and the magnesium connection.

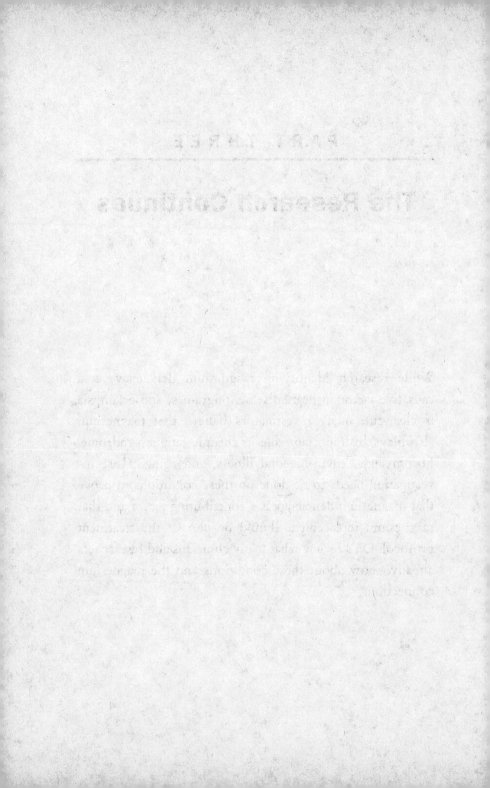

CHAPTER 9

Chronic Fatigue Syndrome and Fibromyalgia

THREE THINGS YOU NEED TO KNOW ABOUT MAGNESIUM, CHRONIC FATIGUE SYNDROME, AND FIBROMYALGIA

1. Magnesium deficiency is common in most chronic fatigue syndrome and fibromyalgia sufferers.
2. Magnesium forms an important part of treatment for chronic fatigue syndrome and fibromyalgia.
3. Magnesium ameliorates the fatigue, muscle pain, and chemical sensitivity of chronic fatigue syndrome and fibromyalgia.

CHRONIC FATIGUE SYNDROME

Over the past one hundred years, we have had a tremendous love affair with chemicals and electronics and a strange marriage with scientific methodology. It is safe to say that important advances in chemicals, pharmaceuticals, and science in general came out of the World War II effort and space research. The unseen potential risks to the public were presumably outweighed by the crisis of the time.

However, our sedentary lifestyle, consumption of synthetic foods, environmental chemicals, and polluted atmosphere have coincided with a greater frequency of chronic fatigue syndrome and fibromyalgia. On a parallel track, magnesium and other nutrients have become woefully depleted and, as we saw in Chapter 4, leave us unable to protect our bodies and brains from chemicals.

Chronic fatigue syndrome (CFS) was formally recognized and defined as an illness by the Centers for Disease Control (CDC) in 1988. Before that time, and even since, many doctors considered the condition psychological. CFS goes by various names: Epstein-Barr, yuppie flu, and, in Britain, myalgic encephalomyelitis (which identifies the muscles and brain as sites of inflammation). Unfortunately, chronic fatigue syndrome is the name that has stuck in the United States, which makes it seem related to the generalized fatigue that anyone can suffer at one time or another. The name minimizes the global impact that this devastating disease can have on a person's life.

The symptoms of CFS are chronic headaches, swollen glands, periodic fevers and chills, muscle and joint aches and pains, muscle weakness, sore throat, and numbness and tingling of the extremities. The general feeling is one of incredible fatigue and inability to do even the simplest of tasks without becoming exhausted, inability to cope with any stress, and insomnia.

There are many theories about the cause of CFS, but one triggering factor could be a reactivation of an already present mononucleosis-like virus called Epstein-Barr virus. Upward of 90 percent of the population already has antibodies to Epstein-Barr virus, meaning the virus infected them at some point in their lives. In most people the infection came and went like a normal cold or flu. But for some, the first infection or the reactivation of the virus can be quite severe and leave them feeling fatigued, run-down, and never truly healthy again.

If CFS is some type of infection presenting itself in a new way, then the people it affects most severely seem to be more run-down and stressed than average. It appears that this infection becomes chronic because the immune system is not strong enough to fight it off or because sufferers come in contact with a chemical or pollutant that undermines their resistance and allows them to succumb to the illness. One of the ways the immune system is stressed is by the generalized depletion of minerals and vitamins that it needs to function properly.

Sheila fit the profile of chronic fatigue syndrome. After

CHRONIC FATIGUE SYNDROME
DIAGNOSTIC CRITERIA

MAJOR CRITERIA

- New onset of fatigue, causing a 50 percent reduction in activity for at least six months
- Exclusion of other illnesses that can cause fatigue

MINOR CRITERIA

- Presence of eight of eleven symptoms, or six of eleven symptoms and two of the three signs

Symptoms

- Mild fever
- Recurrent sore throat
- Painful lymph nodes
- Muscle weakness
- Muscle pain
- Prolonged fatigue after exercise
- Recurrent headache
- Migratory joint pain
- Neurological or psychological complaints: sensitivity to bright light, forgetfulness, confusion, inability to concentrate, excessive irritability, depression
- Sleep disturbance
- Sudden onset of symptom complex

Signs

- Low-grade fever
- Sore throat without signs of pus
- Palpable or tender lymph nodes

having had mononucleosis during college, she had never felt quite the same. The mono seemed to weaken her immune system and her adrenal glands. She worked as a teacher and was constantly exposed to germs, coming down with every cold and flu that passed through the school. Because she traveled a lot, she received numerous inoculations, which further weakened her. In her spare time she enjoyed furniture refinishing, which exposed her to tung oil, found in varnishes, paint strippers, and paint. It is made from euphorbia, a plant that produces phorbol esters, and has been proposed as a causative agent for chronic fatigue syndrome.[1]

After a trip to the Far East, Sheila became more and more fatigued and came down with a terrible monthlong flu with a horribly achy head, muscles, and joints. Her doctor put her on one antibiotic after another, even though she had no bacterial infection. Her cough and chest pain finally cleared up, but she continued to have periodic fevers, a sore throat, and sore muscles. She couldn't exercise at all because she would end up in bed for days, and no matter how tired she was, she couldn't sleep. Sheila was depressed by this constant sickness. Sometimes she felt as if she were losing her mind:

She couldn't concentrate, remember, or perform simple arithmetic. She couldn't teach and was so exhausted that she could do only the bare minimum to take care of herself.

Fortunately, Sheila's doctor was involved with a study at a local university looking into possible drug treatments for CFS. She entered the blind study and did not know which treatment she was receiving. The three medications were an anti-inflammatory drug (ibuprofen), an antidepressant (amitriptyline), and magnesium glycinate. She had weekly visits with a nurse to assess her symptoms, twenty-four-hour urine collections, blood tests, and questionnaires. After two weeks her fatigue improved, as did her muscle weakness, twitching, poor concentration, and irritability.

At the end of the study, Sheila was told that her treatment had been 300 mg of elemental magnesium twice a day, that her magnesium had been very low at the beginning of the study, and that she could safely continue with the treatment if she wished. Sheila now had the energy to do more things to take care of herself: exercise, shop for the right foods, and prepare more meals from fresh foods. She knew she was on the road to recovery, thanks to magnesium. Several other studies confirm the efficacy of using magnesium for the treatment of chronic fatigue syndrome symptoms.[2,3,4,5]

FIBROMYALGIA

It wasn't until 1990 that the American College of Rheumatology established diagnostic criteria for fibromyalgia, there-

FIBROMYALGIA DIAGNOSTIC CRITERIA

MAJOR CRITERIA
- Generalized aches or stiffness of at least three anatomical sites for at least three months
- Six or more typical, reproducible tender points, called trigger points, in the muscles
- Exclusion of other disorders that can cause similar symptoms

MINOR CRITERIA
- Generalized fatigue
- Chronic headaches
- Sleep disturbances
- Neurological and psychological complaints
- Joint swelling
- Numbness or tingling sensation
- Irritable bowel syndrome
- Variation of symptoms in relation to activity, stress, and weather changes.

by giving it official status as an illness. *Fibro-* means "connective tissue" and refers to the thin tissue that wraps around muscles, and *myalgia* means "muscle pain." Also called fibrositis, fibromyalgia is a close cousin of CFS and shares many of its symptoms: incapacitating fatigue, muscle and joint pain, neuralgia, sleep disorders, anxiety, depression, cognitive confusion, and digestive problems. (CFS sufferers, in addition, have mild fever, swollen glands, and a sore throat, which distinguishes them from fibromyalgia patients.) Having a name, however, does not define the causes of the illness, and the American College of Rheumatology does not offer a curative treatment.

I believe fibromyalgia is the latest label for an accumulation of toxins and infections from both environment and lifestyle. Twenty-six doctors who present their cases in a book on chronic fatigue and fibromyalgia agree.[6]

Our exposure to toxins, chemicals, and prescription drugs begins at birth. Substances we think are safe can break down our immune systems and deplete our nutrient reserves. I and many other doctors believe they lead to CFS, fibromyalgia, and environmental illness in a growing list of sufferers.[7] Here's a chronology of ailments and the kinds of treatments any one of us may receive over the course of a lifetime. Each treatment can trigger the next event and further drug intervention.

- Diaper rash, caused by *Candida albicans* (yeast), is treated with cortisone creams, which encourage further growth of the yeast.
- Childhood ear infections can begin at birth as yeast infections picked up from the mother during delivery. Most ear infections are treated with antibiotics.
- Infections may become chronic and require multiple

courses of antibiotics, leading to diarrhea and intestinal yeast infections and irritable bowel.

- Anesthetics used in surgery to place tubes in the ears add another toxin.
- Colic can develop due to antibiotics.
- Inability to digest milk due to an irritated bowel leads to frequent changes of formula and further irritation.
- Gas and bloating can result from hard-to-digest soy formula.
- Eczema, aggravated by food sensitivity, is suppressed with cortisone creams.
- Allergies to foods, especially yeast, wheat, and dairy, can arise from poor digestion.
- Asthma, which may be environmental, is treated with medications including cortisone inhalers.
- Multiple colds and flus are treated with many courses of antibiotics and annual flu vaccines.
- Cravings for sweets can be caused by yeast overgrowth and may cause or aggravate hyperactive behavior in children.
- Dental cavities lead to multiple mercury amalgam fillings. Toxic mercury vapor may be inhaled, absorbed, or disrupt enzymes in the brain, kidneys, and liver.
- Allergic reactions are treated with allergy shots, antihistamines, and cortisone sprays.
- Many adolescents take long-term oral antibiotics for acne.

- Many teens and young adults develop mononucleosis, and up to 20 percent never feel quite as healthy again.
- Bladder infections are treated with antibiotics, which cause yeast infections.
- Birth control pills cause chronic vaginal yeast infections, which are treated with antibiotic creams.
- Pregnancy hormones encourage vaginal yeast infections.
- Chronic sleep deprivation is common in all parents of small children and is a major stress on the immune system.
- Irritable bowel can develop after a bout of diarrhea (attributed to traveler's diarrhea or food poisoning) and is usually treated with antibiotics.
- Hypothyroidism with body temperature below 98.2 degrees F often occurs but remains undiagnosed and untreated.
- Hospitalization for infections or surgery usually warrants intravenous antibiotics and a host of other drugs.
- Major colds and flus can lead to bronchitis and pneumonia, which are treated with strong antibiotics.
- Chronic fatigue syndrome and fibromyalgia are treated with anti-inflammatories, sleeping pills, and antidepressants.
- Environmental allergies with extreme sensitivities to inhalants, especially perfumes, colognes, household products, pesticides, and molds, are treated with cortisone.
- Dysmenorrhea, irregular periods, infertility, and wors-

ening premenstrual symptoms occur due to a buildup of toxins and lack of nutrients.

- Infertility is treated with an array of synthetic hormonal drugs.
- Depression, anxiety, panic attacks, and palpitations are treated with antidepressants and psychotherapy.
- Menopause is medicated with synthetic hormones.

Magnesium is depleted with every step of this scenario and results in a total body burden of drugs, toxins, and various stressors. The end result looks very much like chronic fatigue syndrome.

Let's look at the journey through life from the ground up to understand why we have become so nutrient-deficient and how this affects the immune system.

Plants grown on devitalized, overworked soil that has been poisoned by acid rain are poor in nutrients, including magnesium. Synthetic foods created by modern processing and refining are devoid of natural vitamins, minerals, and fiber. They are "fortified" with useless synthetic vitamins and often no minerals except calcium or iron. Magnesium is the nutrient hardest hit by food processing.

The body is not able to process junk food, with its dozens of chemical additives, in the same way as it does organic food. It treats these chemical additives like foreign invaders and has to detoxify them in the liver. The intermediary metabolites are sometimes more toxic than the original, leaving the body hypersensitive and hyperimmune, sometimes turning on the body and creating autoimmune disease (MS, rheumatoid arthritis). Magnesium is depleted in the attempt to detoxify the body of these foreign chemicals.

There are thousands of medicinal drugs currently in use. Magnesium expert Mildred Seelig tells us that the side effects of many drugs may be associated with magnesium deficiency because magnesium becomes depleted while the body is trying to detoxify these drugs.

With the advent of antibiotics and the hope that they could cure all our infectious diseases, there is an overuse of these powerful drugs. When antibiotics kill bacteria, they cannot discriminate; they kill both good and bad bacteria. The good bacteria killed in the gastrointestinal tract are then replaced with yeast *(Candida albicans)*.

The birth control pill, with its daily hormone surge, feeds yeast in the gut, as do sugar products. Yeast overgrowth results in episodes of alternating diarrhea and constipation. Magnesium is lost due to diarrhea and is drained by the constant demand to balance the pH of the body due to the acidity of soda pop and junk food.

The symptoms from yeast and its breakdown products are bodywide. Often these symptoms lead one to think that there are infections in the sinuses, throat, bladder or vagina. A doctor will consequently prescribe more antibiotics for these symptoms, which perpetuates the problem in a vicious cycle.

Acidity in the intestines from overgrowth of yeast can irritate the intestines to the point of causing micropunctures in their lining, thus allowing the absorption of incompletely digested food into the bloodstream. This food is now a foreign body, and the immune system reacts by forming antibodies to try to get rid of these foreign substances. Food allergies and sensitivities result. Magnesium is one of the minerals in the body that is responsible for neutralizing excess acidity.

Allergies are created when inhaled chemicals and toxins irritate the mucous membranes of the nasal passages. They can trigger symptoms of asthma, which is made worse by magnesium deficiency.

Depression can be a direct result of accumulating chemicals in the body from drugs, synthetic food, and infections. When the brain is deficient in magnesium it is no longer protected from the onslaught of chemicals such as aspartame and MSG.

Because there are no medical tests to confirm that chemicals, drugs, and synthetic food are causing our symptoms, people who feel sick are often told that "everything is normal." This is frustrating and depressing, which makes sufferers feel even more unwell. The majority of chronically ill patients who came to my office had seen between six and thirty doctors in one year for their complaints. Patients with fatigue or depression had usually been referred to a psychiatrist. Some patients had been prescribed thousands of dollars' worth of drugs annually to treat their multiple complaints, which usually did no good and merely added to their toxic load.

The complex nature of CFS and fibromyalgia is formidable. Even though more doctors understand and accept the existence of CFS, the focus of CFS research seems to be on finding one cause. And the treatment is symptomatic: Rheumatologists and psychiatrists treat sleeplessness with sleeping pills; pain with anti-inflammatory drugs, painkillers, and muscle relaxants; and anxiety and depression with anti-anxiety drugs and antidepressants. No attention is paid to diet or nutrient deficiencies. They ignore the possibility that there could be a nutrient imbalance, such as a magnesium deficiency, or coexisting conditions, such as a yeast infection, low thyroid, or allergies, that cause a complex of symptoms. They also tend to overlook possible toxicities, which allow common infections to appear more virulent as they take advantage of a weakened host. Yet magnesium deficiency is known to exacerbate all the symptoms of CFS and fibromyalgia, and it has been effective in helping to restore health to many sufferers. Magnesium is also one of the best ways to strengthen the immune system and boost resistance against germs.

Exercise is often suggested for people suffering from fatigue, but rigorous aerobic exercise is exhausting to people with CFS or fibromyalgia, who have no energy because their magnesium-driven energy system is bankrupt. Exercise also causes lactic acid buildup, which leads to more pain when it is not cleared by a particular enzyme that requires magnesium. Even the work of metabolizing pain medications depletes magnesium. This explains why chronic fatigue patients do not do well on most medications.

A buildup of lactic acid in the muscles causes pain and can be treated with 300 mg of elemental magnesium twice a day. If the joints accumulate toxicity, arthritis can occur; if the nerves are irritated by neurotoxins, they begin to lose their myelin sheath, and MS can result. In fact, autoimmune disease may also be the end stage of a buildup of toxicity along with a deficiency of nutrients, such as magnesium, that are designed to clear toxins from the body. According to some doctors, the definition of autoimmune disease as "disease against self" is not accurate; the disease process is, in fact, against a self altered by toxins and nutrient deficiencies.

Patients with fibromyalgia also have chronically low levels of serotonin, which greatly exaggerates their pain. As mentioned previously, magnesium is a necessary building block for both the production and uptake of serotonin by brain cells.

STRESS

Acute episodes of CFS and fibromyalgia are often brought on by exposure to stress, whether emotional or physical. The consequent increase in adrenaline and stress chemicals hastens magnesium loss and can be a factor in both these conditions. Low levels of magnesium intensify the secretion of the stress chemicals, thus increasing the risk of adverse effects of stress and creating another vicious cycle.[8]

FATIGUE

The overproduction of adrenaline due to stress leads to magnesium deficiency and therefore puts a strain on the magnesium-dependent energy system of the body, causing energy depletion that leads to fatigue. Fatigue is often reduced with magnesium supplementation. In fact, a major breakthrough occurred in CFS research when low magnesium levels were discovered in most sufferers. Of the many enzyme systems that require magnesium, the most important ones are responsible for energy production and storage.

Magnesium and malic acid, an acid found in apples, are both crucial to the body's energy production and useful in the treatment of CFS and fibromyalgia. In the case of fibromyalgia, low magnesium keeps muscles in a state of spasm, so supplementation can aid in relieving this painful symptom. A study by Guy D. Abraham, M.D., showed positive results in the reversal of fibromyalgia with magnesium and malic acid supplementation. Fifteen patients with fibromyalgia who took magnesium (300–600 mg) and malic acid (1,200–2,400 mg) experienced improvement in their symptoms within the first forty-eight hours. Over an eight-week period of supplementation their degree of muscle tenderness and pain dropped from 19.6 points to 6.5 points, according to standardized medical scores.[9]

CHAPTER 10

Environmental Illness and Asthma

> **THREE THINGS YOU NEED TO KNOW ABOUT MAGNESIUM AND ENVIRONMENTAL ILLNESS**
>
> 1. Symptoms of chemical sensitivity can be completely or partially produced by magnesium deficiency.
> 2. Magnesium helps detoxify toxic chemicals.
> 3. Magnesium helps eliminate heavy metals from the body.

Dr. Sherry Rogers is a diplomate in family practice, allergy-asthma-immunology, and environmental medicine and a fellow of the American College of Nutrition. In private practice for more than thirty years, she treats very ill people from all over the world who have environmental toxicity.

One of her basic maxims is that "symptoms of chemical sensitivity can be wholly or in part produced by magnesium deficiency." She has tested enough people over the decades to know this to be a fact and part of her success derives from implementing magnesium therapy on all her patients.

CFS and fibromyalgia are actually aspects of environmental illness. In Chapter 9 we saw how these conditions develop over time in a toxic environment. Now we will take a closer look at some environmentally sensitive people and the chemicals they encountered.

Natalie, sometimes in jest but more often in anger, would call what she experienced a "chemical warfare attack." It happened when she stepped out onto her driveway and was enveloped by a cloud of chemical spray from a lawn care truck treating her neighbor's yard. She could neither breathe nor speak. Her lungs were on fire, and her head felt as though it were exploding. She felt dizzy and shaky. She managed to stagger into the house, where she collapsed on the floor. Her husband found her a few minutes later and took her to the hospital, where they could do very little except give her oxygen and tell her to rest.

Natalie had been the picture of health, athletic, active, and happy. Now she was chronically fatigued. She became hypersensitive to every chemical she came in contact with. She couldn't even read; magazines and newspapers reeked of ink. Perfume samples that came in magazines were a nightmare. She had to find natural substitutes for cleaning products and cosmetics. Plants with moldy-smelling dirt had to go. She became allergic to wool. Her husband had to do all the cooking because she was sensitive to the gas fumes from their stove. Her diet became increasingly limited, as she reacted to many foods. When she couldn't even use the telephone because holding the plastic receiver gave her hives, she became a prisoner in her own home with no contact with the outside world.

Elizabeth, Ted, and their children developed an array of symptoms after they used urea formaldehyde insulation in their home renovation. As soon as it was installed, they noticed an odor. The contractor said not to worry, it would be gone in a few days. The only thing that was gone in a few days was the contractor. They phoned and phoned, but he never returned their calls. By the end of the week the whole family had what appeared to be a bad cold, their eyes and noses streaming. The children developed skin rashes, and they all were irritable, headachy, and tired. When the "cold" didn't go away in ten days they went to the doctor, who saw their red, irritated skin and mucous membranes but no signs of infection, except for swollen neck glands. The doctor suggested they might be allergic to something. That clinched it; they knew it was the insulation. They didn't know what they could do about it. They tried toughing it out to see if the chemical would dissipate, but when the heat came on the next month the problem actually got worse. They were beginning to be allergic to more and more things, and none of them felt well at all. Finally, they decided to rip out all the insulation, no matter what it cost.

Natalie, Elizabeth, Ted, and the children eventually got better. With much time, effort, and money and the help of sympathetic and knowledgeable health practitioners who understand the effects of the environment and the need to detoxify and nourish the body, they regained their health. The modalities they used were pure water, fresh air, organic foods, rotation diets, sauna therapy, vitamin and mineral supplements (especially 300 mg of elemental magnesium twice a day), homeopathy, acupuncture, and a positive attitude.

Some people with the above conditions are not as fortunate as Natalie, Elizabeth, and Ted, who at least knew what was harming them almost from the start. Those who gradually build up allergies and sensitivities to environmental toxins never know they're getting sick until they've developed asthma, eczema, or even cancer. What follows is an overview of our chemical environment and how its impact on our health can be lessened by neuroprotectants like magnesium.

Toxic chemicals were found in nearly all foods tested by the FDA at a level causing a health concern. They included persistent organic pollutants (POPs) such as DDT and dioxin, which have been banned in the United States for decades but are still produced in other countries. Exposure to minuscule levels of POPs at crucial times in fetal and infant development can disrupt or damage human hormone, reproductive, neurological, and immune systems.[1]

In 2000 the Centers for Disease Control released the very first large-scale national survey of environmental toxins from human samples, and the results are startling. Blood and urine levels of twenty-seven chemicals tested in five thousand Americans far exceeded safe levels. The EPA and CDC mostly rely on air, water, and soil samples to test for toxic levels of chemicals. Even then, only a few dozen of the more than one hundred thousand chemicals in everyday use are monitored for safety.[2] Perhaps this human study will reinforce a cutback in chemical pesticide use as pledged by the U.S. Department of Agriculture (USDA) and the U.S. Environmental Protection Agency (EPA) in 1993. Chemical pesticide use, however, has increased from 900 million pounds in 1992 to 940 million pounds in 2000, while total cropland has decreased. And the riskiest chemical pesticides, such as organophosphates, carbamates, probable or possible carcinogens, still account for over 40 percent of the pesticides used in U.S. agriculture.[3]

The average American household generates fifteen pounds of household hazardous waste each year, according to the Texas Natural Resource Conservation Commission. "Our homes contain an average of three to eight gallons of hazardous materials in kitchens, bathrooms, garages and basements," the government agency reports. And what is the consequence of all these chemicals in our home environment? In a California study the number of people with sensitivities to one or more common chemicals is "surprisingly large," according to researchers. Just over 6 percent of the subjects reported having a diagnosis of multiple chemical sensitivity or environmental illness, and nearly 16 percent reported being allergic or unusually sensitive to everyday chemicals.[4]

In 1989, the World Health Organization took a strong stand regarding the origins of cancer when it stated that up to 80 percent of cancers are environmentally influenced. In 1985, the U.S. Environmental Protection Agency published a survey of human fat composition. It found that more than 99 percent of the population had measurable levels of the nine chemicals they tested for, including PCBs and DDT. In 2000, 100 percent of fat samples tested were positive for chemicals. Dr. Samuel Epstein, professor of occupational and environmental medicine at the University of Illinois Medical Center, Chicago, is an internationally recognized authority on the toxic and carcinogenic effects of environmental pollutants in air, water, and the workplace. His research was key to banning DDT and other problematic ingredients and contaminants in consumer products—food, cosmetics, and household products. In his keynote address to a Health Canada–sponsored cancer conference, he reported that we all now carry more than five hundred different compounds in our cells, none of which existed before 1920, and that "there is no safe dose for any of them."[5] With this information, activists have been demanding more use of safe alternatives to chemicals. But government and industry are still not listening.

Chemicals can destroy or paralyze different enzymes that protect us from external toxins. Thus, being exposed to chemicals prevents the body from protecting us from those very chemicals. Magnesium is active in more than 325 enzyme systems in the body, and when its enzymes are paralyzed, it is unable to do its essential work of energy production, detoxification, and brain and nerve protection.

METALS AND MAGNESIUM

Dr. Deborah Baker has researched the health effects of mercury for over a decade.[6] She acknowledges that mercury pervades our environment through industrial exposure, but the major source of elemental mercury in the general North American population is mercury vapor released from dental amalgams.[7,8,9,10] These amalgams are, on average, 50 percent mercury, and they off-gas or vaporize into your body's cells every time you chew, brush your teeth, or eat anything hot or acidic. There is a significant positive correlation between the number of amalgams in the mouth and the mercury content of human tissues, including the brain.[11]

Mercury drastically increases the excretion of magnesium and calcium from the kidneys, which may be caused by the kidney damage seen in mercury poisoning.[12] Such mineral loss impairs cell production, the storage and utilization of energy, and cellular repair and replication. Sufficient magnesium supplementation can not only undo some of this damage but can prevent certain types of heavy metal toxicity.[13,14]

Long-term fetal exposure during pregnancy to even low concentrations of mercury can lead to irreversible developmental disorders.[15] The concentration of magnesium in the placental and fetal tissues necessarily increases during pregnancy.[16] Unfortunately, the demand for magnesium usually exceeds its supply, and thus anything that further lowers magnesium levels, such as mercury, puts the pregnancy and child at risk.

Dr. Baker says that approximately 85 percent of her patients, as part of their mercury detoxification protocol, supplement with 300 mg to 500 mg daily of magnesium glycinate, in divided doses. Patients frequently comment that their muscular pain improves while on magnesium.

Lead and cadmium have a cumulative toxicity on the kidney and heart in particular. Magnesium appears to be a competitive inhibitor of these two polluting metals at different sites, particularly during combined intoxication.[17] A Yugoslavian research team found that increased intake of magnesium eliminates lead via the urine and may do the same with certain other heavy metals. Under experimental conditions, they found that magnesium increased excretion of cadmium via the urine.[18] Adequate magnesium levels can also help prevent the toxic effects of aluminum, which include breakdown of sugar stores and disruption in the production of ATP energy.[19]

TREATMENT

The hallmark of a mineral-deficient person is often one who takes vitamins without minerals and feels worse or does well for a while but then deteriorates.[20] If you have a mineral deficiency, especially of magnesium, which is necessary for energy production, certain areas of the body may be overstimulated by vitamin supplements, while other areas can't respond. Therefore, if you suffer severe environmental illness, it is important to have a health care practitioner monitor supplement intake and to begin with magnesium as one of your first supplements.

The treatment for environmental illness is individualized. Since allopathic medicine does not recognize environmental disease, it has not established treatment protocols. According to environmental experts, magnesium is essential to build up the body's energy and fully utilize its detoxification systems. The source of environmental toxins, however, must be eliminated or avoided; otherwise it is like bailing out a sinking ship by hand. You first have to be aware of the chemicals in your environment, avoid them like the plague, and work diligently with the therapies that follow to clean out your body.

The lowly dry cleaning chemicals, the mercury in dental fillings, and the cleaning products under the sink all build up in our bodies and cause chronic disease. Air purifying machines, water filters, organic food, organic supplements, and natural alternatives to chemicals provide the foundation of environmental health treatment.

DIET

The key in treating environmental illness is to eat organic, free-range, unprocessed, unadulterated foods. The pesticides added to the soil and the antibiotics used on poultry and beef sicken the animals and the people who eat them. The rash of diseases in cattle is likely related to the low quality of their feed, the tons of drugs they are given to fatten them up, and the gallons of chemicals sprayed on them to treat parasites. Unfortunately, even organic farms are subjected to acid rain, contaminated groundwater, and polluted air, which means that all of us should take an active role in detoxifying our bodies of suspected chemicals.

Drink six to eight glasses of pure water a day. Chemicals in our environment that are water-soluble are eliminated through the kidneys and colon, especially if you drink enough pure water. Use a filter that has a pore size of less than 0.5 microns and guarantees the elimination of chemicals as well as parasites.

To eliminate fat-soluble chemicals such as pesticides and herbicides, which can become even more toxic when they are broken down by the liver, you need dry saunas and sea clay wraps. Fasting is not recommended to eliminate toxins. Fat-soluble chemicals are stored in fat cells, which keeps them out of circulation. When you try to fast or diet, your fat stores are broken down for energy, and out come the chemicals. The headache, nausea, light-headedness, and irritability are not just from lack of food but from poisons flooding your bloodstream. While fasting, I've tasted and felt the numbing effect of dental anesthetics from decades before. If you are already feeling ill, fasting and dieting are going to be very unpleasant experiences.

DRY SAUNA

Numerous cultures use sweat lodges, steam baths, or saunas for cleansing and purification. Many health clubs and big apartment buildings have saunas and steam baths, and more and more people are building saunas in their own homes. Low-to-moderate-temperature saunas are one of the most important ways to detoxify from pesticide exposure. Head-to-toe perspiration through the skin, the largest organ of elimination, releases stored toxins and opens the pores. Fat that is close to the skin is heated, mobilized, and broken down, releasing toxins and breaking up cellulite. The heat increases metabolism, burns off calories, and gives the heart and circulation a workout. This is a boon if you don't have the energy to exercise. It is well known in medicine that a fever is the body's way of burning off an infection and stimulating the immune system. Fever therapy and sauna therapy are employed at alternative medicine healing centers to do just that. The controlled temperature in a sauna is excellent for relaxing muscular aches and pains and relieving sinus congestion. The only way I made it through my medical internship was by having regular saunas to reduce the daily stress.

SEA CLAY WRAPS

A very appealing method of detoxification is the Universal Contour Wrap. In Europe it is promoted as a healing and cleansing modality; however, in America it can be marketed only as a beauty treatment. It is an extremely safe and effective method of detoxification. A licensed technician uses large tensor bandages soaked in liquid clay to wrap your whole body from toe to neck. The process draws out poisons, toxins, and edema. Measurements before and after the hourlong treatment show actual loss of inches. The health and appearance of the skin is much improved. It even works to eliminate cellulite. You can obtain a kit to do your own partial wraps. See the Resources section for more information.

SUPPLEMENTS

If you have environmental illness, you feel as though you are sensitive or allergic to everything. When it comes to taking supplements, you may be unable to tolerate anything, but you might be deficient in everything. This does not necessarily mean that you are allergic to a particular supplement; rather, when you take it, your body responds by increasing some metabolic processes, which results in the body throwing off waste products that make you feel nauseous or headachy. That is why an organic diet, saunas, sea clay wraps, and exercise should be implemented before taking supplements.

The first supplement to add is magnesium. Start with 100 mg of elemental magnesium once a day and add a second capsule after a week, a third in the third week, and a fourth a week later, in divided doses. Cut back if you have loose stools. "Green drinks" are the next food supplement to add. They are made from a variety of organic land and sea vegetables and flavored with stevia. Some "green drinks" are made with whey protein powder and make a good cleansing drink or meal replacement for a modified fast.

By now you should be feeling much better and able to add some more supplements to help boost your immune system and provide necessary building blocks for health. Environmental illness does not require high-dose supplementation like other diseases. In fact, since most megavitamins and minerals are derived synthetically, it is a far better approach to use low-potency food-based supplements from organic sources. Standard Process supplements, for example, meet these criteria and are available from natural health practitioners, who can assist you in developing an individualized program.

MAGNESIUM AND ASTHMA

As a child, Gerry had eczema. Every possible skin cream and lotion was tried, to no avail, but finally, after many years, the last patch disappeared on its own. It was followed almost immediately, however, by his first asthma attack. By age thirty, he was suffering attacks of wheezing and coughing when he exercised and when he was around cats, dogs,

**THREE THINGS YOU NEED TO KNOW
ABOUT MAGNESIUM AND ASTHMA**

1. Research shows that many patients with asthma and other bronchial diseases have low magnesium.
2. Many drugs used in the treatment of asthma cause a loss of magnesium, making symptoms only worse.
3. Patients treated with simple magnesium supplementation report marked improvement in their symptoms.

horses, dust, flowers, and chemical smells. Various medications helped initially, but after a year or two they would stop working. He wasn't satisfied with them, anyway; one gave him heart palpitations, and another contained cortisone, which made him gain weight and retain fluid. Then one day a vitamin newsletter came in the mail. He almost threw it out, but a headline caught his attention: "Magnesium Halts Asthma Spasms."

Asthma is characterized by bronchial spasm, swelling of the mucous membranes of the lung, excessive mucus production, and an inability to fully empty the lungs of air. Asthma finds its easiest victims in children under ten and is twice as common in boys and men, although it affects about 3 percent of the general population. Tabulating all the triggers of an asthma attack is a daunting task; there seems to be a variety of stimuli, including lung infection, exercise, emotional upset, food sensitivities, inhalation of cold air or irritating aromatic substances (smoke, gas fumes, paint fumes, chemical fumes), and reactions to specific allergens, such as pollens.

Bronchial spasms occur in both extrinsic asthma (an allergic reaction to external substances such as mold, dust, animal hair, pollens and chemicals) and intrinsic asthma (from exercise, infection, and emotional upset). The allergic triggers, called allergens, initiate the release of histamines in your body, which try to eliminate the allergens by stimulating lots of mucus to mop up the allergens and push them out through sneezing, coughing, and watery eyes. One of the side effects of too much histamine is tightening of the bronchial tubes, which go into spasm. Such spasms can initiate episodic wheezing, coughing, and shortness of breath, which quickly lead to rapid breathing, difficulty exhaling, anxiety, and dehydration. The anxiety of an asthma attack can create a gripping fear that tenses up the whole body and is hard to shake off.

Gerry really identified with what he read about asthma and magnesium, and he realized that his whole body was tense. He decided to try some magnesium supplements under his doctor's supervision, and with them he was able to greatly decrease his medications.

Magnesium is an excellent treatment for asthma because it is a natural antihistamine and a bronchodilator. It has a calming effect on the muscles of the bronchial tubes and the whole body. Certainly, drug therapy for asthma can often be lifesaving; drugs, however, are not curative. You have to eliminate the underlying cause of asthma and replace magnesium to fully treat this condition. Without magnesium, asthma can become chronic, especially if the various triggers are not eliminated; even the fear of an attack can magnify the emotional component. Conventional allergy shots have been used for decades to try to trick the body into accepting irritating allergens but often do not work, especially when the condition is due to a nutrient deficiency.

According to Dr. Seelig, the drug treatment of asthma consists of magnesium-wasters such as beta blockers, cortisone, and ventolin. The side effects of these drugs include severe magnesium deficiency that can result in arrhythmia and sudden death.[21] Theophylline (Aminophylline) results in loss of magnesium and suppression of vitamin B_6 activity, which is necessary for magnesium function. Prednisone wastes magnesium, causes sodium retention and fluid retention, suppresses vitamin D, and causes increased urinary excretion of zinc, vitamin K, and vitamin C.[22]

Childhood asthma can be life-threatening; but safe methods of treating this condition can be added. In a European study, a group of children who had deteriorated in spite of conventional drug therapy were given magnesium sulfate intravenously. Comparing the magnesium group with the placebo group, the magnesium group had lower clinical asthma scores and a significantly greater percentage of improvement in lung function over a ninety-minute period. No significant side effects were observed.[23]

Dr. Lydia Ciarallo in the Department of Pediatrics, Brown University School of Medicine, treated thirty-one asthma patients ages six to eighteen who were deteriorating on conventional treatments. One group was given magnesium sulfate and another group was given saline solution, both intravenously. At fifty minutes the magnesium group had a significantly greater percentage of improvement in lung function, and more magnesium patients were discharged from the emergency department than the placebo group who went on to hospitalization.[24]

Another study showed a correlation between intracellular magnesium levels and airway spasm. The investigators found that patients who had low cellular magnesium levels had increased bronchial spasm. This finding confirmed not only that magnesium was useful in the treatment of asthma by dilating the bronchial tubes but that lack of magnesium was probably a cause of this condition.[25]

A team of researchers identified magnesium deficiency as surprisingly common, finding it in 65 percent of an intensive-care population of asthmatics and in 11 percent of an outpatient asthma population. They supported the use of magnesium to help prevent asthma attacks. Magnesium has several antiasthmatic actions. As a calcium antagonist, it relaxes airways and smooth muscles and dilates the lungs. It also reduces airway inflammation, inhibits chemicals that cause spasm, and increases anti-inflammatory substances such as nitric oxide.[26]

The same study established that a lower dietary magnesium

intake was associated with impaired lung function, bronchial hyperreactivity, and an increased risk of wheezing. The study included 2,633 randomly selected adults ages eighteen to seventy. Dietary magnesium intake was calculated by a food frequency questionnaire, and lung function and allergic tendency were evaluated. The investigators concluded that low magnesium intake may be involved in the development of both asthma and chronic obstructive airway disease.

DIET

Avoid sugar. Limit red meat and dairy, which contain substances that increase inflammation in the body. Increase yellow vegetables and green leafy vegetables, which contain substances that inhibit inflammation. Increase intake of fish oils, seed and nut oils, cold-water fish (herring, sardines, salmon), flaxseed oil, and walnuts to reduce inflammation. Eat grapes; grape skins contain quercetin, which prevents histamine release and inhibits inflammatory products.

Try a liquid fast: Use a therapeutic whey protein powder, a green drink, and/or fresh, organic juices plus fiber for three days, followed by a vegetarian diet for four days.

Get out of the rut of eating the same foods every day and eliminate possible food allergies. Eggs, shellfish, and peanuts usually cause immediate sensitivity reactions; milk, chocolate, wheat, citrus, and food colorings cause delayed food reactions. Carefully check labels in the grocery store and speak up in restaurants to avoid even small amounts of potential allergic triggers.

Avoid aspirin and nonsteroidal anti-inflammatories (e.g., ibuprofen), which can cause allergic reactions.

Clean out environmental allergies: Find other homes for cats and dogs. Avoid wall-to-wall carpeting, wall hangings, and feather pillows. Frequently replace or clean air filters for heating and cooling systems. Obtain environmentally sound cleaning products. Use a vacuum cleaner specific for allergies. Research HEPA air cleaners and ozone generators.

SUPPLEMENTS

Magnesium: 300 mg twice a day

Vitamin B_6: 50 mg twice a day

Pantothenic acid: 500 mg daily

Vitamin C: 1–2 g daily

Vitamin E as mixed tocopherols: 400 IU daily

Quercetin: 500 mg three times a day

Selenium: 250 mcg a day

Flaxseed oil: 1–2 tbsp daily

Hydrochloric acid: 5 grains, 1 tablet per day at the end of a meal, increasing to one with each meal.

CHAPTER 11

Health and Longevity

THREE THINGS YOU NEED TO KNOW
ABOUT MAGNESIUM AND AGING

1. Magnesium is deficient in people who have Alzheimer's disease or Parkinson's disease.
2. Aging itself is a risk factor for magnesium deficiency; as we get older we become more deficient in magnesium and therefore require more in our diet and in supplement form.
3. Magnesium binds and eliminates toxic chemicals and metals to keep them from contributing to symptoms of aging.

Three hundred years ago, people didn't live as long as we do today. They lived in such unsanitary conditions that simple scrapes and cuts became mortal wounds. Bathing was looked upon with suspicion. Tuberculosis, fostered by extremely close quarters, little sun exposure, lack of fresh vegetables, and dampness, was highly contagious and struck down many in their prime. Indoor fires without adequate ventilation made for chronic bronchitis and emphysema, if the people even lived long enough to develop these conditions.

When we implemented universal sanitation, the infectious diseases began to recede. The land was still fertile, and plants soaked up vital nutrients. Farm animals ate them, and humans absorbed them from eating fresh meat and fresh produce. The industrial revolution, however, harmed our health in a new way, with factories belching smoke and chemical poisons. Industrial farming techniques began poisoning the soil with pesticides, herbicides, and nitrogen fertilizers. The soil became lifeless.

We may think we are better off in this century with our drugs and medical technology, but as we've seen, these can also become toxic and undermine our health, especially in a polluted environment where our basic nutrition is impaired. Popping antiaging pills and megavitamins do *not* add years to your life. An excellent diet that provides optimal nutrients, exercise, and an outgoing, optimistic attitude are the true keys to longevity.

Aging in industrialized societies is associated with an

increasing prevalence of hypertension, heart disease, reduced insulin sensitivity, and adult-onset diabetes. Aging in general is associated with altered calcium and magnesium ion levels, indistinguishable from those observed in hypertension and diabetes.[1] In Chapters 5 and 6 we talked about insulin resistance and its role in exacerbating hypertension, heart disease, and diabetes mellitus. Insulin-resistant states, as well as what is often thought of as "normal" aging, are characterized by the accumulation of calcium and depletion of magnesium in the cells. With all this in mind, clinical researchers suggest that it is the disturbance of calcium and magnesium ions that might be the missing link responsible for the frequent clinical coexistence of hypertension, atherosclerosis, and metabolic disorders in aging.[2]

As evident from animal experiments and epidemiological studies, magnesium deficiency may increase our susceptibility to cardiovascular heart diseases as well as accelerate

"Smart drugs" such as piracetam, oxiracetam, pramiracetam, and aniracetam are thought to enhance learning, facilitate the flow of information between the two hemispheres of the brain, help the brain resist physical and chemical injuries, and supposed to be free of side effects. Magnesium fits all the criteria for "smart drugs," but it is much less costly and has no side effects.

aging.[3] In a study on nursing home residents, low magnesium levels were significantly associated with two conditions that plague the elderly, calf cramps and diabetes mellitus.[4] Centenarians (individuals reaching a hundred years of age) have higher total body magnesium and lower calcium levels than the usual elderly person.[5]

FREE RADICALS, ANTIOXIDANTS, AND AGING

A free radical is an unstable molecule that is the product of normal body metabolism. It is formed when molecules within our own body's cells react with oxygen. It has an unpaired electron that tries to steal a stabilizing electron from another molecule and as a consequence can produce harmful effects. External sources of free radicals include chemicals (pesticides, industrial pollution, auto exhaust, cigarette smoke), heavy metals (dental amalgam, lead, cadmium), most infections (viruses, bacteria, parasites), X rays, alcohol, allergens, stress, and even excessive exercise.

Antioxidants are vitamins and minerals such as magnesium, selenium, vitamin C, and vitamin E that turn off free radicals. The greater the amount of other antioxidants in the body, the more magnesium is spared from acting as an antioxidant and is free to perform its many other functions. So antioxidants protect the level of magnesium in the body, which prevents elevation of calcium, which can lead to vascular muscle spasm.[6] If there are not enough antioxidants available, overabundant free radicals begin to damage and destroy normal, healthy cells. Free radicals are necessary and normal products of metabolism, but uncontrolled free radical production plays a major role in the development of degenerative disease, since free radicals can damage any body structure: proteins, enzymes, fats, even DNA. Free radicals are implicated in more than sixty different health conditions, including heart disease, autoimmune disease, and cancer.

According to current research, low magnesium levels not only magnify free-radical damage but can hasten the production of free radicals.[7] One study utilizing cultures of skin cells found that low magnesium doubled the levels of free radicals.[8] In addition, cells grown without magnesium were twice as susceptible to free radical damage as were cells grown in normal amounts of magnesium. Another study showed that red blood cells from hamsters fed low-magnesium diets were deficient in magnesium and consequently more susceptible to free-radical damage. It appears that low magnesium damages the vital fatty layer in the cell membrane, making it more susceptible to destruction and allowing leakage through the membrane.

A number of reports have identified pesticides as a cause of Parkinson's disease (which affects over one million Americans), with in-home exposure to insecticides carrying the highest risk.[9] Glutathione is a naturally occurring antioxidant made in all the cells of the body, including neurons, which acts to detoxify the body of certain chemicals. Cells grown in magnesium-deficient conditions, however, have lower glutathione levels. Adding free radicals to a low-magnesium cell culture causes glutathione levels to fall rapidly, making the cells much more susceptible to free radical damage. Neurosurgeon Dr. Russel Blaylock tells us that a fall in cellular glutathione within part of the brain called the substantia nigra appears to be one of the earliest findings in Parkinson's disease.[10]

ALZHEIMER'S

In North America, approximately 10 percent of the population over sixty-five, and 50 percent over eighty-five, suffer from Alzheimer's. It is associated with severe memory loss, impaired cognitive function, and inability to carry out activities of daily life. Alzheimer's disease is often diagnosed when all the other identifiable brain conditions are ruled out (e.g., brain tumor, alcoholism, vitamin B_{12} deficiency, mercury amalgam poisoning, depression, hypothyroidism, Parkinson's, stroke, excessive prescription drug use). In truth, it is only at autopsy that a definitive diagnosis can be made. The brain will show the identifying characteristics of Alzheimer's: plaques and tangles in the nerve fibers, particularly in the cerebrocortex and hippocampal area. Dr. Abram Hoffer, the founder of orthomolecular medicine along with Linus Pauling, cautions that almost half the diagnosed cases of Alzheimer's may be such treatable conditions as simple dehydration, prescription drug intoxication, severe cerebral allergies to foods or chemicals, or chronic nutrient deficiencies.

Chemicals and toxic metals are associated with Alzheimer's disease, especially aluminum, which many Americans are exposed to through aluminum pots, aluminum cans, aluminum-containing antacids and antiperspirants, aluminum foil, and tap water that may be high in aluminum.[11,12] Considerable research has proven that brain neurons affected in Alzheimer's disease have significantly higher levels of aluminum than normal neurons. Alzheimer's patients also have consistently low magnesium levels within the hippocampus, the area of the brain most damaged by Alzheimer's. Aluminum is able to replace magnesium in certain enzyme systems in the body, mimicking its function but causing harm. Aluminum can also replace magnesium in the brain, which leaves calcium channels in the brain nerve cells wide open, allowing calcium to flood in, causing cell death.[13]

PARKINSON'S DISEASE

Similarly, with Parkinson's disease aluminum can be a contributing factor in central nervous system degeneration. In one autopsy study, calcium and aluminum were elevated in the brains of victims of Parkinson's disease as compared to people with normal brains.[14]

Enzymes function in the body only when they have access to the proper cofactors, which are mostly vitamins and minerals, especially magnesium, selenium, vitamin C, vitamin B_6, and vitamin E. Heavy metals such as cadmium, aluminum, and lead attach themselves to certain enzymes, kicking out minerals such as magnesium, and either prevent the normal enzyme activity or create abnormal activity leading to cell destruction.

Research indicates that ample magnesium will protect brain cells from the damaging effects of aluminum, beryllium, cadmium, lead, mercury, and nickel. We also know that low levels of brain magnesium contribute to the deposition of heavy metals in the brain that heralds Parkinson's and Alzheimer's. It appears that the metals compete with magnesium for entry into the brain cells. If magnesium is low, metals gain access much more readily.

There is also competition in the small intestine for absorption of minerals. If there is enough magnesium, aluminum won't be absorbed. When monkeys are fed diets low in calcium and magnesium but high in aluminum, for instance, they become apathetic and begin to lose weight. When their spinal cords are examined under the microscope, they show swelling of the anterior motor cells (movement centers), plus accumulation of calcium and aluminum in these cells.[15] If you eat from aluminum pots, use aluminum-containing antiperspirants, wrap your food in aluminum foil, and drink tap water with high aluminum content, the levels could overwhelm the magnesium in your gut, and aluminum will be absorbed instead. This has consequences on the amount of magnesium in your brain and allows the buildup of aluminum associated with Alzheimer's and Parkinson's disease.

It may be that aluminum acts as a co-toxin in these diseases, adding to the toxicity produced by excitotoxins.

Dr. Blaylock reports that when scientists study the soil of regions that have a high incidence of neurological diseases, they find high levels of aluminum and low levels of magnesium and calcium. The neurons from victims of the disease also show high levels of aluminum and low levels of magnesium. On the island of Guam the areas with the lowest levels of calcium and magnesium in the soil are also the areas of highest incidence for all neurological diseases. Magnesium plays a vital role in protecting neurons from the lethal effects of aluminum.[16]

William Grant, an atmospheric scientist, had an interest in Alzheimer's because of a strong family history. Grant already knew that people with Alzheimer's typically have elevated concentrations of aluminum in their brains. He put that bit of information together with the fact that acid rain makes aluminum more abundant in trees and seems to make trees age prematurely. Grant theorized that the diets of Alzheimer's patients might be very acidic, leaching the calcium and magnesium from the body. He found that people with Alzheimer's have elevated amounts of aluminum, iron, and zinc and have reduced amounts of alkali metals such as magnesium, calcium, and potassium, which neutralize the acidity in the diet. An acid-forming diet is the typical Western fare—high protein, high fat, and high sugar are additional factors in creating aluminum overload in Alzheimer's.

The body's ability to absorb magnesium declines with

age, so at particular risk are elderly people who do not eat an adequate diet and who use drugs that deplete the body's magnesium. (Studies show that senior citizens take on average six to eight medications regularly.) Add to that the effects of antacids, which many elderly people take to cover up symptoms caused by a bad diet. Antacids suppress normal stomach acid and can lead to incompletely digested food, which causes gas, bloating, and constipation. Another hidden danger is the use of aluminum in most antacids.

But aside from the direct toxic effect of aluminum, dementia may also be caused by magnesium depletion alone.[17] Several studies show that severe neurological syndromes can result when conditions cause extremely low levels of brain magnesium, such as with the chronic use of diuretics, which millions of people take to control high blood pressure. These neurological conditions can present as seizures, delirium, coma, or psychosis, which are quickly reversed by administering large doses of intravenous magnesium. Excessive amounts of aspartame and MSG (glutamate) in the diet of elderly people may also cause symptoms of dementia due to their direct effect, which is also magnified in magnesium deficiency.

Dr. Jean Durlach, a preeminent magnesium expert in France, sums up the current research on magnesium and aging.[18]

1. Chronic marginal magnesium deficiency reduces life span in rats.
2. Magnesium deficiency accelerates aging through its

various effects on the neuromuscular, cardiovascular, and endocrine apparatus; kidneys and bones; and immune, antistress, and antioxidant systems.

3. In developed countries, magnesium intake is marginal throughout the entire population regardless of age: around 4 mg/kg/day instead of the 6 mg/kg/day recommended to maintain satisfactory balance. However, the elderly population is extremely heterogeneous: diseases, handicaps, and physical or psychological impairments expose individuals to more severe nutritional deficiencies.

4. Around the age of seventy, magnesium absorption becomes two-thirds of what it is at age thirty.

5. Various mechanisms of deficiency include intestinal malabsorption; reduced bone uptake and mobilization (osteoporosis); increased urinary losses; chronic stress; insulin resistance leading to diabetes with severe magnesium loss in the urine; lack of response to adrenal stimulation; loss caused by medication, especially diuretics; alcohol addiction; and cigarette smoking.

6. Magnesium deficiency symptoms in the elderly include central nervous system symptoms that seem largely "neurotic": anxiety, excessive emotionality, fatigue, headaches, insomnia, light-headedness, dizziness, nervous fits, sensation of a lump in the throat, and impaired breathing. Peripheral nervous system signs are common: pins and needles of the extremi-

ties, cramps, muscle pains. Functional disorders include chest pain, shortness of breath, chest pressure, palpitations, extra systoles (occasional heart thumps from an isolated extra beat), abnormal heart rhythm, and Raynaud's syndrome. Autonomic nervous system disturbances involve both the sympathetic and parasympathetic nervous systems, causing hypotension on rising quickly or borderline hypertension. In elderly patients, excessive emotionality, tremor, weakness, sleep disorders, amnesia, and cognitive disturbances are particularly important aspects of magnesium deficiency.

7. A trial of oral magnesium supplementation is the best diagnostic tool for establishing the importance of magnesium.

TREATMENT BEYOND MAGNESIUM

MANAGEMENT OF ALUMINUM TOXICITY
AND ALZHEIMER'S

Use only filtered water that guarantees removal of aluminum; drink eight glasses per day. Check labels and avoid antacids containing aluminum. Use natural antiperspirants. Avoid cooking in aluminum pots or drinking fruit juice or soft drinks from aluminum containers. Get checked for thyroid disease and treat appropriately. Check for heavy metal toxicity (aluminum, mercury, copper, lead, and iron) through urine testing or hair analysis. Pursue either oral or intravenous chelation to remove your heavy-metal burden.

DIET

Avoid all junk food and salty, fried, and fatty foods. Stay away from meat, alcohol, coffee, caffeine, and sugar. Check for food sensitivities, particularly wheat and dairy. Therapeutic foods include cilantro, onion, seaweeds and ginger, which help bind and excrete heavy metals.

SUPPLEMENTS

Magnesium: 300 mg two or three times per day

Calcium: 500 mg twice per day

Vitamin E as mixed tocopherols: 400 IU daily

Vitamin C: 1,000 mg twice per day

B complex: 50 mg twice per day

Vitamin B_{12}: 1,000 mcg intramuscularly weekly

Lecithin granules: 2 tbsp per day

Flaxseed oil: 1–2 tbsp per day

Fish oil (halibut liver oil or cod liver oil): 1 tsp per day

In addition, the herbs *Ginkgo biloba* and *Gota cola* improve cerebral circulation. Drugs that worsen Alzheimer's include chlorpromazine, antihistamines, barbiturates, psychotropic drugs, and diuretics.

ALTERNATIVE THERAPIES FOR ALZHEIMER'S

Avoid mercury fillings or have them replaced. But the work must be done by a dentist who specializes in this area; improper removal can result in more mercury being released into the tissues. Clean out all the chemicals in your home and immediate environment. Eat organic food. Exercise and take regular saunas.

PART FOUR

Testing and Supplements

CHAPTER 12

Magnesium Requirements, Testing, and Sources

MAGNESIUM REQUIREMENTS

The Recommended Daily Allowance (RDA) for nutrients is set at the minimum level to stave off deficiency symptoms, not at the maximum that ensures good health. But even with the RDA set so low, most Americans are still deficient in magnesium.

The following table shows the Recommended Daily Allowances (RDAs) for magnesium in children and adults.

Children 1 to 3 years: 80 mg
Children 4 to 8 years: 130 mg
Children 9 to 13 years: 240 mg

Life Stage	Men	Women	Pregnancy	Lactation
Age 14–18	410 mg	360 mg	400 mg	360 mg
Age 19–30	400 mg	310 mg	350 mg	310 mg
Age 31+	420 mg	320 mg	360 mg	320 mg

The RDA for magnesium is also expressed in mg/kg and is roughly 6 mg per kg (2.2 lbs) of body weight. This standard helps to determine the magnesium requirements for someone who is overweight, because a fifty-year-old who weighs 300 pounds needs more magnesium than a fifty-year-old who is 100 pounds.

Many magnesium experts feel that the RDA should be increased. Twenty years of research shows that under ideal conditions approximately 300 mg of magnesium is required merely to offset the daily losses. If you are under mild to moderate stress caused by a physical or psychological disease, physical injury, athletic exertion, or emotional upheaval, your requirements for magnesium escalate.[1,2] Dr. Mildred Seelig feels that adolescent boys and girls who are athletic may need 7–10 mg/kg/day and pregnancy requirements should be a minimum of 450 mg a day or up to 15 mg/kg/day.[3] An average diet may supply about 120 mg of magnesium per 1,000 calories, for an estimated daily intake of about 250 mg.[4,5] Since at best the body is actually absorbing only half of what is taken in, researchers feel that most people would benefit from magnesium supplementation. Otherwise, body tissue must be broken down to supply vital areas of the body with essential magnesium.[6,7]

MAGNESIUM TESTING

You've heard the saying "To err is human, to forgive is divine"? In the medical world, to err is human, to test is divine.

Laboratory tests should be used to confirm what our senses and intuition tells us, but all too often doctors place all their faith in tests. Yet finding the definitive test for a condition, which can clinch a diagnosis, makes both doctor and patient feel safe. Over the years lab testing for minerals evolved from measurements done on whole blood to isolating minerals inside cells. The present state of the art, however, lies in testing mineral ions, which are the active component of minerals working at the tissue level.

There are two clinical tests that can be done in a doctor's office, the results of which can indicate both calcium deficiency and magnesium deficiency: Chvostek's sign (a contraction of the facial muscles caused by tapping lightly on the facial nerve located in front of the ear) and Trousseau's sign (a spasm of the hand muscles caused by applying a tourniquet or blood pressure cuff to the forearm below the elbow for three minutes). But since neither test distinguishes calcium deficiency from magnesium deficiency, doctors use the test to diagnose and treat only calcium deficiency. As a result, magnesium levels are driven even lower, causing more symptoms.

TOTAL SERUM (BLOOD) MAGNESIUM TEST

In spite of, or perhaps because of, all the metabolic processes that rely on magnesium, less than 1 percent of our body's total magnesium can be measured in our blood; the rest is busily occupied in the cells and tissues. Therefore, it is virtually impossible to extrapolate and make an accurate assessment of the level of magnesium in various body tissue cells using a routine total serum magnesium test. Magnesium in the blood does not correlate with the amount of magnesium in other parts of your body. In fact, if you are under the stress of various ailments, your body pumps magnesium out of the cells and into the blood, giving the mistaken appearance of normality on testing in spite of bodywide depletion. Unfortunately, most magnesium evaluations done in hospitals and in laboratories use this antiquated total serum magnesium test.

RED AND WHITE BLOOD CELL MAGNESIUM TESTS
All body cells, including red and white blood cells, contain up to 40 percent of the body's magnesium. Studies show that red blood cell magnesium is a somewhat more accurate measure of total body magnesium than the total serum magnesium test. One study in childhood asthmatics compared total serum magnesium levels to total white blood cell magnesium levels. While total serum magnesium became elevated on the first day of an asthma attack, the total white blood cell magnesium levels dropped dramatically, indicating the real state of affairs. As mentioned above, under stress magnesium is released from the cells, depleting them, as it floods into the bloodstream.[8] However, total red blood cell and total white blood cell magnesium levels are not as accurate measures of the actual tissue levels of magnesium as are ionized magnesium levels in cells, which we will dicuss later.

THE MAGNESIUM CHALLENGE TEST

Time-consuming and cumbersome, the magnesium challenge test requires two twenty-four-hour urine collections. The first collection is done while the patient is taking his or her normal supplements. Then, in the doctor's office, a dose of 2 meq/kg of magnesium chloride or magnesium sulfate is given intravenously, infused over a four-hour period. A second urine collection begins after the IV and is continued for twenty-four hours. Deficiency is diagnosed when the body exhibits a need for magnesium by holding on to more than 25 percent of the magnesium given. A decade ago, the magnesium challenge test was the best method of determining body stores.[9] However, comparison studies using magnesium challenge and ionized magnesium indicate that ionized magnesium testing appears to be a better indicator and more easily done (see next page).[10]

THE BUCCAL SMEAR

One innovative test, which is not readily available, is the buccal cell smear test. A scraping is taken from the mucous membranes on the floor of the mouth under the tongue. The total mineral levels in the buccal cells correlate with the results from white blood cells and red blood cells. Analysis is performed using scanning electron microscopy (SEM) and elemental X-ray analysis (EXA). Once again, when compared with ionized magnesium testing, the buccal smear comes up short because this test is measuring total cellular magnesium contents, as are the red blood cell and white blood cell tests. It is not measuring active, free magnesium ions.

BLOOD IONIZED MAGNESIUM TEST

The blood ionized magnesium test, pioneered and tested extensively at the State University of New York in Brooklyn by magnesium researchers Bella and Burton Altura, is the most accurate and reliable magnesium blood test available. The Alturas have researched the health effects of magnesium since the 1960s and did the original research for the test in 1987.[11,12,13,14,15,16]

The ionic magnesium test is a very refined procedure, backed up by results on many thousands of patients with over twenty-two different disease states and published in dozens of journals, including five papers in *Science* and papers in the prestigious *Scandinavian Journal of Clinical Laboratory Investigation* and *Scientific American*.[17] To determine the efficacy and efficiency of the new test, research included a comparison of magnesium levels found with the Alturas' ionized magnesium test to levels found in various body tissues using expensive and sensitive digital imaging microscopy, atomic absorption spectroscopy, and the magnesium fluorescent probe. The blood ionized magnesium test came through as a highly sensitive, convenient, and relatively inexpensive means of determining magnesium status in healthy or ill subjects.

Here's how it works. Magnesium exists in the body either as active magnesium ions or as inactive magnesium complexes bound to proteins or other substances. A magnesium ion is an atom that is missing two electrons, which makes it search to attach to something that will replace its missing electrons. Magnesium ions constitute the physiologically active fraction of magnesium in the body; they are not attached to other substances and are free to join in biochemical body processes.[18]

Most clinical laboratories assess only *total* serum magnesium, which includes both active and inactive types. With the blood ionized magnesium test it is now possible to directly measure the levels of magnesium ions in whole blood, plasma, and serum using ion-selective electrodes.[19]

For example, ionized magnesium testing on three thousand migraine patients shows that 90 percent of those with low magnesium ion levels improve with magnesium therapy. In 85 to 90 percent of all patients tested, low magnesium ion levels match tissue levels of free magnesium and accurately diagnose magnesium deficiency found in asthma, brain trauma, coronary artery disease, types I and II diabetes, gestational diabetes, eclampsia and preeclampsia, heart disease, homocysteinuria, hypertension, tension headaches, posttraumatic headaches, ischemic heart disease, liver transplant patients, renal transplant patients, polycystic ovarian disease, stroke, and syndrome X. In many of these conditions, low magnesium ion levels exist in spite of normal total serum magnesium levels, making the ionized magnesium test more reliable for magnesium deficiency diagnosis.[20,21,22,23,24,25,26,27,28,29]

The FDA-approved ionized magnesium test is being ordered by more and more doctors as they become familiar with the dozens of research papers confirming its efficacy. The testing continues to be performed in a handful of labs, including the Alturas' laboratory, with blood samples coming in from all over the United States.[30] A few years back a spate of testing in some research labs using inferior electrodes produced inferior results. The Alturas, therefore, will provide the test to doctors for a fee and at the same time help other clinical labs set up the right protocol and equipment to do their own ionized magnesium testing properly. (See the Resources section for further information on the ionized magnesium test.)

THE ORAL CLINICAL TRIAL

For the average individual, who does not have easy access to the ionized magnesium test, one way to diagnose magnesium deficiency is simply to try supplementing. For one to three months take magnesium while recording all changes in your physical and mental health. It may be best to do this under a health professional's guidance, especially if you are on medications or have an existing medical condition. The alleviation of symptoms after thirty to ninety days constitutes the best proof that you had a magnesium deficiency.

See "Magnesium Supplements," page 228, for types of magnesium and dosage.

FALSE-POSITIVE MAGNESIUM TESTS

The lack of adequate tools to measure magnesium in most hospitals and clinics is another reason medical doctors do not prescribe it. A total serum magnesium test is actually worse than ineffective, because a test result that is within normal limits lends a false sense of security about the status of the mineral in the body. It also explains why doctors don't recognize magnesium deficiency; they assume total serum magnesium levels are an accurate measure. Magnesium researchers mostly use total serum and total red blood cell magnesium tests to determine magnesium status. As they begin to use the more accurate ionized magnesium test, however, the results will indicate even more widespread deficiency in the population.

DIET SOLUTIONS TO
MAGNESIUM DEFICIENCY

Good nutrition creates a solid foundation of tissue and bone. The basis of good nutrition is the consumption of minerals, trace minerals, vitamins, amino acids, and essential fatty acids. Clearly there is more to life than magnesium, but life can't exist without it.

To enrich your diet with magnesium, increase your

consumption of green vegetables, nuts, seeds, legumes, and unprocessed grains. Removing the germ of cereals and the outer seed husks through processing eliminates most of the magnesium present in the whole grain. It is a good idea to supplement a diet of fruit and protein-rich foods such as fish, meat, and milk by eating wheat germ, kelp, brewer's yeast, sunflower seeds, pumpkin seeds, and sea salt, which are all extremely rich in magnesium. Since one of the reasons you may be magnesium-deficient is from eating too much cooked food, try to eat more raw foods. Fortunately, nuts, seeds, and many vegetables can be eaten raw, and raw wheat germ can be used on cereal and in protein drinks.

According to top French magnesium experts, highly effective heart- and blood vessel–protective diets that reduce saturated fats, increase monounsaturated fat and omega-3 fatty acids (from fish and flaxseed), limit the consumption of alcohol, and increase the intake of cereals, fruits, vegetables, fish, and low-fat dairy products that are rich in magnesium. They stress that among several protective nutrients, magnesium should be given particular consideration because of the very frequent occurrence of chronic primary magnesium deficiency, which acts as a cardiovascular risk factor.[31]

ORGANIC FOOD

Factory-farmed food is deficient in magnesium; therefore, organic food is a wiser choice. As more people go this route, whether to avoid herbicide and pesticide residues or to ensure nutrient-dense produce, the cost of organic food is dropping dramatically. However, organic food is not a guarantee of higher magnesium levels. Seek out organic farmers who are educated about crop rotation, test regularly for mineral deficiencies in the soil, and use mineral-rich fertilizers. The smart way to be assured of quality organic food is to join a community-sponsored agriculture (CSA) cooperative and buy a share in a local organic farm every year. Every week for an average of twenty-four weeks you share the harvest, which can include fresh vegetables, fruit, and free-range eggs, chicken, and lamb. (See the Resources section for contact information on CSAs.)

USDA FINDINGS

The United States Department of Agriculture (USDA) surveys of women's diet find that approximately 25 percent of their magnesium is supplied by grain products. This means you should try to include a variety of whole grains and avoid refined white bread and pasta. (If you crave sugar and bread, you might be addicted to carbohydrates and should try to limit your intake to achieve weight loss and blood sugar balance.) Another 25 percent of magnesium intake comes from fruits and vegetables. The high-protein foods—meat, poultry, and fish—provide only about 18 percent of total magnesium intake. Since protein diets are now becoming more popular, you must make sure to increase your intake of magnesium when on such a diet. Fats, sweets, and beverages supply 14 percent of the total magnesium intake; however, these foods, especially refined fats and sweets, should be limited because they contain empty calories devoid of nutrients. Natural fats from nuts and seeds and their butters are the richest sources of magnesium, but they are not even mentioned in most food surveys.

MAGNESIUM SOURCES

In the Appendix you will find a complete list of foods with their magnesium content. Here is a short list of the richest sources of magnesium.[32] The quality of the soil from which these sources were assayed is unknown. Therefore, use these figures as a rough guide to making magnesium-wise food choices.

MAGNESIUM CONTENT OF SELECTED FOODS

(mg per 3½ oz [100 g/10 tbsp] serving)

Kelp	760
Wheat bran	490
Wheat germ	336
Almonds	270
Cashews	267

Molasses	258
Yeast, brewer's	231
Buckwheat	229
Brazil nuts	225
Dulse	220
Filberts	184
Peanuts	175
Wheat grain	160
Millet	162
Pecan	142
English walnuts	131
Rye	115
Tofu	111

HERB SOURCES OF MAGNESIUM

Green plants, including most herbs, like purslane and cilantro, are loaded with magnesium.[33,34,35,36] Here are some other commonly used magnesium-rich herbs that you can introduce into your diet. Herbs have the added advantage of being mostly organic or picked wild, so they usually don't contain pesticides and herbicides.

BURDOCK ROOT (ARCTIUM LAPPA) 537 MG MAGNESIUM PER 100 G

Master herbalist Matthew Wood describes burdock root as a diuretic for kidney gravel, an excellent blood cleanser, and a liver detoxifier. It can be grated into salads or cooked like potato and eaten several times per week.

CHICKWEED *(STELLARIA MEDIA)* 529 MG MAGNESIUM PER 100 G

Herbalist Susun Weed describes chickweed as a perfect food with "optimum nutrition." Chickweed encourages absorption of minerals and nutrients and is also naturally high in magnesium. Used several times a week in salads, it provides an excellent source of dietary magnesium.

DANDELION *(TARAXACUM OFFICINALE)* 157 MG MAGNESIUM PER 100 G

This amazing herb has been vilified as a nuisance weed, but its healing properties are legion. According to Andrew Chevallier, an experienced medical herbalist, it is used as a diuretic to treat high blood pressure, and as a detoxifier removing waste products from the gallbladder and the kidneys, thereby ameliorating many conditions such as gallstones, constipation, acne, eczema, arthritis, and gout. No doubt it owes some of its actions to the properties of magnesium. Dandelion leaves, used in salads, add a necessary bitter property that stimulates the bile. The root can be cooked or grated raw into salads.

DULSE *(PALMARIA PALMATA)* 220 MG MAGNESIUM PER 100 G

There are many forms of dulse or seaweed, and all are very nutritional. They are very high in digestible protein, around 25 percent by weight. Iodine to support the thyroid gland is their most notable benefit. They are high in most minerals as well as vitamins. Dulse can be introduced several times a week in soups and stews, and don't forget vegetarian sushi rolls, which are wrapped in seaweed.

NETTLES *(URTICA DIOICA)* 860 MG MAGNESIUM PER 100 G

Nettles are used to soften gallstones or kidney stones in the body. Susun Weed has some excellent recipes for nettles in her book *Healing Wise*. When nettles are lightly steamed they lose their stinging properties and make an excellent vegetable addition to any meal.

MINERAL WATER AND MAGNESIUM

An important source of magnesium, popular in Europe, is magnesium-rich mineral water. We have only a few local waters in the United States that have high magnesium levels that could help to reduce magnesium deficiency. We must also be careful to consider the calcium content of bottled water in relation to magnesium. A close reading of labels tells us that calcium and sodium are usually much higher than magnesium. Therefore, choose water with calcium no more than twice the level of magnesium. This will ensure that you are getting enough of both minerals. If, however, you know you have a magnesium deficiency, by symptoms or by medical or naturopathic diagnosis, choose water with high magnesium and low calcium content for replacement. And if you suffer from heart disease, choose mineral water with low sodium content. Be aware that even though a label says "mineral water," the mineral contents may be minuscule and not worth the price you pay.[37]

MAGNESIUM IN WATER[38]

Water Name	Country	Magnesium (mg/L)	Calcium (mg/L)	Sodium (mg/L)
Adobe Springs	USA	96	3.3	5
Santa Ynez	USA	87	19	—
San Pellegrino	ITALY	57	203	46
Penafiel	MEXICO	41	131	159
Vittel	FRANCE	38	181	3.7
Evian	FRANCE	24	78	5
Naya	CANADA	22	38	6
Volvic	FRANCE	7	10	10.7
Saratoga	USA	7	64	9
Perrier	FRANCE	5	143	15.2
Alhambra	USA	5	9.5	5.4
Arrowhead	USA	5	20	3
Sparkletts	USA	5	4.6	15.2
Calistoga	USA	2	8	163
Cobb Mountain	USA	2	5.6	4.6

Water Name	Country	Magnesium (mg/L)	Calcium (mg/L)	Sodium (mg/L)
Poland Spring	USA	2	13.2	8.9
Sante	USA	1	4.2	160
Black Mountain	USA	1	25	8.3
Crystal Geyser	USA	1	1.5	30

CHAPTER 13

Supplementation and Homeopathics

When you take supplements it can be a real challenge to find out how much actual or elemental magnesium is available in each pill or capsule. Magnesium does not exist alone in nature but comes combined with other substances. That other substance, tagging along with magnesium, has a specific weight. Presently, I take two 500 mg capsules of magnesium oxide, but each capsule does not contain 500 mg of magnesium. Only 60 percent of a magnesium oxide capsule is magnesium; the other 40 percent is the attached oxide. Sixty percent of 500 mg is 300 mg. Of that 300 mg, I may be absorbing only half; half of 300 mg gives me 150 mg. (So, two 500 mg capsules give me a total of 300 mg of magnesium.) My diet supplies another 200 mg, putting me well above the RDA for women, which is 320 mg. Some days, when I am under significant stress, I take three instead of my normal two 500 mg magnesium oxide capsules. When my bowel movements get soft and unformed, I know to go back to two per day. I also switch brands and switch types of magnesium every few months to give my body a change so I don't get used to any one type of magnesium, and to see what works best for me.

There is one more thing to be aware of on product labels, which is the specification of dosage. All too often people will find that they have to take not one but three or six tablets to make up the dosage on the label. It may be in small print, but read it carefully to understand exactly what each tablet contains.

MAGNESIUM DOSAGE

To individualize your magnesium dosage, the rule of thumb for men is 6–8 mg/kg (3.0 to 4.5 mg/lb) of body weight per day. That translates into a total dietary magnesium of 600 to 900 mg per day for a 200-lb man. Some researchers recommend 10 mg/kg/day for children because of their low body weight and increased requirements for growth and 6–10 mg/kg/day for athletes, depending on stress and training levels.[1,2,3,4]

**CONTRAINDICATIONS TO
MAGNESIUM THERAPY**

1. **Kidney failure.** With kidney failure there is an inability to clear magnesium from the kidneys.
2. **Myasthenia gravis.** Intravenous administration could accentuate muscle relaxation and collapse the respiratory muscles.
3. **Excessively slow heart rate.** Slow heart rates can be made even slower, as magnesium relaxes the heart. Slow heart rates often require an artificial pacemaker.
4. **Bowel obstruction.** The main route of elimination of oral magnesium is through the bowel.

THE SAFETY OF MAGNESIUM SUPPLEMENTS

For the average person, oral magnesium, even in high dosages, has no side effects except loose stools, which is a mechanism to release excess magnesium and an indication to cut back. Excess magnesium is also lost through the urine.

TYPES OF MAGNESIUM

Bone meal is a rich source of magnesium. More than 60 percent of the magnesium in the bodies of humans and animals is in the bones and teeth. Since 1945, radioactive strontium 90, along with lead and a variety of other toxic elements, began to show up in our bones and in the bones of cattle from which bone meal is produced. It is important, therefore, to find an organic source of bone meal, strictly assayed for contaminants, if you wish to consume this product. Another reason it makes good sense to use only organic animal products is the possibility of mad cow disease turning up in this country in the future.

Chelated magnesium, bound to organic amino acids, is said to be better absorbed but is more expensive. Complementary medicine practitioners rely on chelated magnesium, such as magnesium glycinate, to treat serious cases of magnesium deficiency.

Weight for weight and dollar for dollar, magnesium oxide may be the best buy for general use.

TYPES OF MAGNESIUM

Inorganic salts	Organic salt chelates
Magnesium oxide	Magnesium glycinate
Magnesium carbonate	Magnesium aspartate
Magnesium chloride	Magnesium glutamate
Magnesium sulfate	Magnesium adipate
Magnesium phosphate	Magnesium citrate
Magnesium bicarbonate	Magnesium orotate
	Magnesium taurate
	Magnesium lysinate

MAGNESIUM CONTENT OF
VARIOUS SUPPLEMENTS

Magnesium Salt	Amount of Elemental Magnesium per 500 mg Salt
Magnesium oxide	300 mg
Magnesium carbonate	150 mg
Magnesium chloride	60 mg
Dolomite	75 mg
Magnesium lactate	60 mg
Magnesium glycinate	50 mg
Magnesium sulfate	50 mg
Magnesium gluconate	25 mg

WHEN TO TAKE MAGNESIUM

I take my first dose of magnesium when I wake up in the morning and the last dose at bedtime. If I take a third dose, that will be in the late afternoon. Magnesium is most deficient in the early morning and late afternoon. Some people feel that magnesium is sufficiently energizing that it keeps them awake at night. Others, who feel it helps their leg cramps, fibromyalgia, or general muscle tension, take it at night and find that it helps them relax and sleep well. There are so many ways that magnesium can work on the body that it is important for you to decide what timing is best for you.

MAGNESIUM AS A LAXATIVE

Oral doses of magnesium sulfate (Epsom salts), magnesium hydroxide (milk of magnesia), and magnesium citrate contain high concentrations of magnesium to draw water into the colon and act as an effective laxative. These salts are, in fact, more gentle than herbal cascara or senna, which cause muscle contraction of the intestinal wall. Laxatives, in general, are not recommended because you can become dependent on them and they can flush out beneficial intestinal bacteria and electrolytes. It is far better to supplement the diet with magnesium-rich foods and, if necessary, magnesium supplements to relax the bowel and allow normal action. Magnesium laxatives are contraindicated in patients with nausea, vomiting, appendicitis, intestinal obstruction, undiagnosed abdominal pain, or kidney disease.

Epsom salts in a bath are absorbed slightly and are known to be relaxing. I remember one patient, Arlene, as "the woman who soaked too long." She put several pounds of Epsom salts in a bath, soaked for two hours, and found out that magnesium sulfate is indeed absorbed through the skin: She developed diarrhea due to magnesium's laxative effect. Someone with a skin condition such as eczema might absorb magnesium even more readily. Limit your soak to forty-five minutes and follow the directions on the label for how much Epsom salts to add to your bath (as a general rule, use no more than 2 cups at a time).

MAGNESIUM SUPPLEMENT ABSORPTION

If you have digestive problems with gas and bloating, which indicates a lack of hydrochloric acid, you may need to take a digestive aid such as betaine hydrochloride to help absorb your minerals. Magnesium can be taken with or without meals, but I prefer to take it between meals for better absorption. Magnesium requires stomach acid to be absorbed. After a full meal, your stomach acid is busy digesting the food and may not be available to help absorb the magnesium. Also, magnesium is an alkaline mineral and acts like an antacid; taken with meals, it may neutralize stomach acid and impair digestion.

If you develop loose stools while taking magnesium, it does not necessarily mean you are absorbing enough and losing the rest; it may mean you are taking too much at one time. Never take your daily magnesium all at once. Spread it out through the day; four times a day is best if you've been experiencing diarrhea. If that doesn't do the trick, you probably need to cut back the amount you're taking or switch to another type or brand of magnesium. Remember that when you first begin taking magnesium, you may need a certain quantity to remedy an existing deficiency; but over time, that deficiency will be eliminated and you might need less. Your stools will tell you. *Note:* If you are taking a multivitamin-mineral supplement, remember to check the amount of elemental magnesium on the label and count it in your daily total.

CALCIUM AND MAGNESIUM INTERACTION

Watch your calcium intake. We know that too much calcium will impede magnesium uptake and function. Push aside the media-generated hype on calcium and look at the facts. A thousand years ago our diet favored magnesium over calcium. Current research seems to indicate that three parts calcium to two parts magnesium is probably most beneficial, with average optimal amounts of calcium at 1,000 mg per day and magnesium at 600 mg.[5]

MAGNESIUM INTERACTION WITH OTHER NUTRIENTS

Magnesium is extremely important for the metabolism of calcium, potassium, phosphorus, zinc, copper, iron, sodium, lead, cadmium, hydrochloric acid, acetylcholine, and nitric oxide, as well as for the activation of vitamin B_1 and therefore for a very wide spectrum of crucial body functions.[6] A shift in any one of these nutrients has an impact on magnesium levels and vice versa. It is the interwoven nature of the body and all its components that makes it so difficult to isolate one substance to scientifically "prove" what it can do. Magnesium cannot be taken out of context either in a research setting or in your body. For example, you should increase magnesium intake when you consume more phosphorus and vitamin D. Magnesium is necessary to convert dietary vitamin D into one of the hormones that makes efficient use of calcium in bone formation.[7,8] Vitamin B_6 increases the amount of magnesium that can enter cells; as a result, these two nutrients are often taken together. In one experiment, serum vitamin E levels improved after magnesium supplementation.[9] We also know that magnesium and the essential fatty acids (EFAs, found in fish, nuts and seeds, and flaxseed oil) are interdependent; each works much more efficiently when the other is present in sufficient amounts.

HOMEOPATHIC MAGNESIUM: ANOTHER FORM OF MAGNESIUM

Developed by Samuel Hahneman in the early nineteenth century, homeopathy is a natural medical science that uses mostly plants and mineral extracts diluted in alcohol or water to infinitesimal amounts in order to stimulate the individual's natural healing response. Research has shown that these medicines, if given in a toxic amount, can cause symptoms similar to those that the patient is experiencing, but that the infinitesimal dose can cure those symptoms. After two hundred years of clinical use and observation, homeopathy is now more successful than the tools we have available to measure how it works. Although skeptics often attribute its success to the placebo effect, in which a patient's belief in an outcome produces that outcome, the millions who have benefited from homeopathy include infants and animals, two groups that are clearly not susceptible to the placebo effect.

Nonetheless, in America homeopathy continues to be marginalized in favor of other drugs, even in the face of such early evidence as the influenza epidemic of 1919, in which the homeopathic hospitals in England showed a greater cure rate than conventional hospitals. In Europe, both homeopathic medicine and herbal medicine enjoy a respected place in the health care system.

Homeopathic remedies typically come in dosages of 6, 12 or 30 X (10) or C (100) potency. The higher the number, the greater the dilution and the more potent the remedy. Usually, you take three pellets or four drops of a remedy several times a day. For a very acute, painful symptom, a dose can be taken every fifteen minutes. However, if after taking five or six doses of a remedy there is no change in symptoms, the remedy is probably ineffective and you should seek a new remedy. Be assured that treating with the wrong remedy a half dozen times does not cause any negative side effects.

In homeopathy, magnesium is used primarily for acute muscle spasms or chronic complaints.[10] Please consult a homeopath for a more detailed evaluation of your case.

MAGNESIA PHOSPHORICA

Magnesia phosphorica (magnesium phosphate, or mag phos) is a great antispasmodic remedy and the most commonly used magnesium homeopathic remedy. It readily treats cramping of all muscles, including hiccups, leg cramps, writer's cramp, abdominal colic, heart pain, lung pain, menstrual pain accompanied by radiating pains, neuralgic pains, and all sorts of tics and tremors including twitching of the eyelids. It works especially well in debilitated subjects who are both mentally and physically tired.

Dr. Margery Mullins, an internist and acupuncturist, recently wrote to tell me about the success she has had with the use of magnesium phosphate (mag phos) for muscle spasms. She said patients would get instant relief and then didn't seem to need the remedy after their magnesium deficiency was corrected with diet and supplements. One of her young patients, a nine-year-old girl, was having such severe muscle spasms that she was referred to a pediatric neurologist. In the interim, Dr. Mullins gave her Magnesia phosphorica 6X, and by the time of her appointment with the specialist the child no longer had the problem. Dr. Mullins noted that the girl's mother had had toxemia (eclampsia) during her pregnancy, requiring intravenous magnesium.

Appendix

MAGNESIUM CONTENT OF SELECTED FOODS

(in mg per 3½ oz [100 g] serving)

Kelp	760
Wheat bran	490
Wheat germ	336
Almonds	270
Cashews	267
Molasses	258
Yeast, brewer's	231
Buckwheat	229
Brazil nuts	225
Dulse	220
Filberts	184

Peanuts	175
Millet	162
Wheat grain	160
Pecan	142
English walnuts	131
Rye	115
Tofu	111
Coconut meat, dried	90
Brown rice	88
Soybeans, cooked	88
Figs, dried	71
Apricots	62
Dates	58
Collard greens	57
Shrimp	51
Corn, sweet	48
Avocado	45
Cheddar cheese	45
Parsley	41
Prunes, dried	40
Sunflower seeds	38
Barley	37
Beans, cooked	37
Dandelion greens	36
Garlic	36
Raisins	35
Green peas, fresh	35
Potato with skin	34

Crab	34
Banana	33
Sweet potato	31
Blackberry	30
Beets	25
Broccoli	24
Cauliflower	24
Carrot	23
Celery	22
Beef	21
Asparagus	20
Chicken	19
Green pepper	18
Winter squash	17
Cantaloupe	16
Eggplant	16
Tomato	14
Milk	13

Resources

IONIC MAGNESIUM TESTING
Drs. Bella and Burton Altura
State University of New York
Health Science Center at Brooklyn
450 Clarkson Avenue
New York, NY 11203
(718) 270-2194 or (718) 270-2205

ORGANIC FOOD
Buy a share in an organic farm in your area.
Join Community Sponsored Agriculture (CSA)
(800) 516-7797
www.reeusda.gov/csa.html

SEA CLAY WRAP

Universal Contour Wrap and Sea Clay
Totally You, Inc.
(800) 458-6549

HOLISTIC MEDICAL ORGANIZATIONS

The American College for Advancement in Medicine
(ACAM)
23121 Verdugo Drive, Suite 204
Laguna Hills, CA 92653
Fax (949) 455-9679
www.acam.org

American Academy of Environmental Medicine
7701 East Kellogg, Suite 625
Wichita, KS 67207
(316) 684-5500
Fax (316) 684-5709
www.aaem.com

American Academy of Pain Management
13947 Mono Way, #A
Sonora, CA 95370
(209) 533-9744
www.aapainmanage.org

American Holistic Medical Association (AHMA)
6728 McLean Village Drive

McLean, VA 22101-8729
(703) 556-9728
Fax (703) 556-8729
www.holisticmedicine.org

American Association of Preventive Medicine
9912 Georgetown Pike, Suite D-2
P.O. Box 458
Great Falls, VA 22066
(800) 230-AAHF
(703) 759-0662
Fax (703) 759-6711
www.apma.net

The Foundation for the Advancement of Innovative
    Medicine (FAIM)
P.O. Box 7016
Albany, NY 12225-0016
(877) 634-3246
Fax (518) 758-7967
www.faim.org

International Society for Orthomolecular Medicine
16 Florence Avenue
Toronto, Ontario, Canada M2N 1E9
(416) 733-2117
Fax (416) 733-2352
www.orthomed.org

Holistic Dental Association
P.O. Box 5007
Durango, CO 81301
www.holisticdental.org

American Association of Naturopathic Physicians
8201 Greensboro Drive, Suite 300
McLean, VA 22102
(703) 610-9037
Fax (703) 610-9005
(877) 969-2267
www.naturopathic.org

International and American Associations of Clinical
    Nutritionists
16775 Addison Road, Suite 100
Addison, TX 75001
(972) 407-9089
Fax (972) 250-0233
www.iaacn.org

American Holistic Nurses' Association
P.O. Box 2130
Flagstaff, AZ 86003-2130
(800) 278-2462
www.ahna.org

References

INTRODUCTION

1. Aikawa JK, *Magnesium: Its Biologic Significance*, CRC Press, Boca Raton, FL, 1981
2. Iannello S, Belfiore F, "Hypomagnesemia. A review of pathophysiological, clinical and therapeutical aspects." *Panminerva Med*, vol. 43, no. 3, pp. 177–209, 2001
3. Altura BM, "Introduction: importance of Mg in physiology and medicine and the need for ion selective electrodes." *Scand J Clin Lab Invest Suppl*, vol. 217, pp. 5–9, 1994
4. Institute of Medicine, *Dietary Reference Intake for Calcium, Phosphorus, Magnesium, Vitamin D, and Fluoride*, National Academy Press, Washington DC, 1997
5. Durlach J, *Magnesium in Clinical Practice*, Libbey, London, 1988
6. Fehlinger R, "Therapy with magnesium salts in neurological diseases." *Magnes Bull*, vol. 12, pp. 35–42, 1990
7. Ducroix T, "L'enfant spasmophile—Aspects diagnostiques et therapeutiques." *Magnes Bull*, vol. 1, pp. 9–15, 1984

CHAPTER 1

1. Altura BM, Altura BT, "Cardiovascular risk factors and magnesium: relationships to atherosclerosis, ischemic heart disease and hypertension." *Magnes Trace Elem,* vol. 92, no. 10, pp. 182–192, 1991

2. Eisenberg MJ, "Magnesium deficiency and sudden death." *Amer Heart J,* vol. 124, no. 2, pp. 544–549, 1992

3. Turlapaty PD, Altura BM, "Magnesium deficiency produces spasms of coronary arteries: relationship to etiology of sudden death ischemic heart disease." *Science,* vol. 208, no. 4440, pp. 198–200, 1980

4. Altura BM, "Sudden-death ischemic heart disease and dietary magnesium intake: is the target site coronary vascular smooth muscle?" *Med Hypotheses,* vol. 5, no. 8, pp. 843–848, 1979

5. Karppanen H et al., "Minerals, coronary heart disease and sudden coronary death." *Adv Cardiol,* vol. 25, pp. 9–24, 1978

6. Rogers SA, *Depression Cured at Last,* SK Publishing, Sarasota, FL, 2000

7. Henrotte JG, "Type A behavior and magnesium metabolism." *Magnesium,* vol. 5, pp. 201–210, 1986

8. Cernak I, et al., "Alterations in magnesium and oxidative status during chronic emotional stress." *Magnes Res,* vol. 13, no. 1, pp. 29–36, 2000

9. Goldberg B, *Alternative Medicine Guide: Women's Health Series 1,* Future Medicine Publishing, Tiburon, CA, 1998

10. Aikawa JK, *Magnesium: Its Biologic Significance,* CRC Press, Boca Raton, FL, 1981

11. Levine BS, Coburn JW, "Magnesium, the mimic/antagonist of calcium." *N Engl J Med,* vol. 310, pp. 1253–1255, 1984

12. Iseri LT, French JH, "Magnesium: nature's physiologic calcium blocker." *Am Heart J,* vol. 108, pp. 188–193, 1984

13. Seelig MS, "Cardiovascular reactions to stress intensified by magnesium deficit in consequences of magnesium deficiency on the enhancement of stress reactions; preventive and therapeutic implications: a review." *J Am Coll Nutr,* vol. 13, no. 5, pp. 429–446, 1994

14. Rodale JR, *Magnesium: The Nutrient That Could Change Your Life,* Rodale Press, Emmaus, PA 1971

15. Hartwig A, "Role of magnesium in genomic stability." *Mutat Research,* vol. 18, no. 475 (1–2), pp. 113–121, 2001
16. Pfeiffer CC, *Zinc and Other Micro-Nutrients,* Keats, New Canaan, CT, 1978
17. Walker GM, "Biotechnological implications of the interactions between magnesium and calcium." *Magnes Res,* vol. 12, no. 4, pp. 303–309, 1999
18. Altura BM, "Sudden-death ischemic heart disease and dietary magnesium intake: is the target site coronary vascular smooth muscle?" *Med Hypotheses,* vol. 8, pp. 843–848, 1979
19. Eades M, Eades A, *The Protein Power Lifeplan,* Warner Books, New York, 1999

CHAPTER 2

1. Kant AK, "Consumption of energy-dense, nutrient-poor foods by adult Americans: nutritional and health implications. The third National Health and Nutrition Examination Survey, 1988–1994." *Am J Clin Nutr,* vol. 72, no. 4, pp. 929–936, 2000
2. Institute of Medicine, *Dietary Reference Intake for Calcium, Phosphorus, Magnesium, Vitamin D, and Fluoride,* National Academy Press, Washington DC, 1997
3. Werbach MR, *Nutritional Influences on Illness,* Thorstons Publishing Group, Wellingborough, Northamptonshire, 1989.
4. Ibid.
5. Eades M, Eades A, *The Protein Power Lifeplan,* Warner Books, New York, 1999
6. Ibid.
7. Worwag M, Classen HG, Schumacher E, "Prevalence of magnesium and zinc deficiencies in nursing home residents in Germany." *Magnes Res,* vol. 3, pp. 181–189, 1999
8. Linderman RD, "Influence of various nutrients and hormones on urinary divalent cation excretion." *Ann NY Acad Sci,* vol. 162, pp. 802–809, 1969
9. Lemann J et al., "Evidence that glucose ingestion inhibits net renal tubular reabsorption of calcium and magnesium in man." *J Lab Clin Medicine,* vol. 75, pp. 578–585, 1970
10. Abbot L et al., "Magnesium deficiency in alcoholism: possible con-

tribution to osteoporosis and cardiovascular disease in alcoholics." *Alcohol Clin Exp Res,* vol. 19, pp. 1076–1082, 1994

11. Barbagallo M, Dominguez LJ, Resnick LM, "Insulin-mimetic action of vanadate: role of intracellular magnesium." *Hypertension,* vol. 3, pt. 2, pp. 701–704, 2001

12. *Physicians' Desk Reference.* 56th ed. Medical Economics, 2002.

13. Ibid.

14. Crossen C, *Tainted Truth: The Manipulation of Fact.* Simon & Schuster, New York, 1995

15. Teo KK et al., "Effects of intravenous magnesium in suspected acute myocardial infarction: overview of randomized trials." *Brit Med J,* vol. 303, pp. 1499–1503, 1991

16. Teo KK, Yusuf S, "Role of magnesium in reducing mortality in acute myocardial infarction. A review of the evidence." *Drugs,* vol. 46, pp. 347–359, 1993

17. Altura BM, "Sudden-death ischemic heart disease and dietary magnesium intake: is the target site coronary vascular smooth muscle?" *Med Hypotheses,* vol. 5, no. 8, pp. 843–848, 1979

18. Altura BM, "Introduction: importance of Mg in physiology and medicine and the need for ion selective electrodes." *Scand J Clin Lab Invest Suppl,* vol. 217, pp. 5–9, 1994

19. Mauskop A, Fox B, *What Your Doctor May Not Tell You About Migraines.* Warner Books, New York, 2001

20. Mauskop A et al., "Deficiency in serum ionized magnesium but not total magnesium in patients with migraines. Possible role of ICa2+/IMg2+ ratio." *Headache,* vol. 33, no. 3, pp. 135–138, 1993

21. Mauskop A et al., "Intravenous magnesium sulphate relieves migraine attacks in patients with low serum ionized magnesium levels: a pilot study." *Clin Sci (Colch),* vol. 89, no. 6, pp. 633–636, 1995

22. Seelig MS, "The requirement of magnesium by the normal adult." *Am J Clin Nutr,* vol. 14, pp. 342–390, 1964

23. Seelig MS, "Cardiovascular reactions to stress intensified by magnesium deficit in consequences of magnesium deficiency on the enhancement of stress reactions; preventive and therapeutic implications: a review." *J Am Coll Nutr,* vol. 13, no. 5, pp. 429–446, 1994

24. Durlach J, *Magnesium in Clinical Practice,* Libbey, London, 1988

25. Durlach J, "Diverse applications of magnesium therapy," in

Handbook of Metal-Ligand Interactions in Biological Fluids—Bioinorganic Medicine, vol. 2, Marcel Dekker, New York, 1995

CHAPTER 3

1. Klerman GL, Weissman MM, "Increasing rates of depression." *JAMA*, vol. 261, no. 15, pp. 2229–35, 1992
2. Weissman MM, "Cross-national epidemiology of major depression and bipolar disorder." *JAMA*, vol. 276, no. 4, pp. 293–9, 1996
3. Murphy JM, "A 40-year perspective on the prevalence of depression: the Stirling County Study." *Arch Gen Psychiatry*, vol. 57, no. 3, pp. 209–215, 2000
4. Michiel RR, "Sudden death in a patient on a liquid protein diet." *New Engl J Med*, vol. 298, pp. 1005–1007, 1978
5. Werbach MR, "Nutritional influences on aggressive behavior," *Journal of Orthomolecular Medicine*, vol. 7, no. 1, 1995
6. Rogers SA, *Depression Cured at Last*, SK Publishing, Sarasota, FL, 2000
7. Durlach J, "Diverse applications of magnesium therapy," in *Handbook of Metal-Ligand Interactions in Biological Fluids—Bioinorganic Medicine*, vol. 2, Marcel Dekker, New York, 1995
8. Seelig MS, "Mechanisms of interactions of stress, stress hormones and magnesium in consequences of magnesium deficiency on the enhancement of stress reactions; preventive and therapeutic implications: a review." *J Am Coll Nutr*, vol. 13, no. 5, pp. 429–446, 1994
9. Cernak I et al., "Alterations in magnesium and oxidative status during chronic emotional stress." *Magnes Res*, vol. 13, pp. 29–36, 2000
10. Classen HG et al., "Coping with acute stress reaction by plentiful oral magnesium supply." *Magnes Bull*, vol. 17, pp. 1–8, 1995
11. Mocci F, Canalis P, Tomasi PA, Casu F, Pettinato S, "The effect of noise on serum and urinary magnesium and catecholamines in humans." *Occup Med (Lond)*, vol. 51, no. 1, pp. 56–61, 2001
12. Starobrat-Hermelin B, Kozielec T, "The effects of magnesium physiological supplementation on hyperactivity in children with attention deficit hyperactivity disorder (ADHD). Positive response to magnesium oral loading test." *Magnes Res*, vol. 10, no. 2, pp. 149–156, 1997
13. Galland L, *Superimmunity for Kids*, Bantam Doubleday Dell, New York, 1988

14. Rogers SA, *Depression Cured at Last,* SK Publishing, Sarasota, FL, 2000

15. Crosby V, Wilcock A, Corcoran R, "The safety and efficacy of a single dose (500 mg or 1 g) of intravenous magnesium sulfate in neuropathic pain poorly responsive to strong opioid analgesics in patients with cancer." *J Pain Symptom Management,* vol. 1, pp. 35–39, 2000

16. Seelig MS, "Athletic stress, performance and magnesium in consequences of magnesium deficiency on the enhancement of stress reactions; preventive and therapeutic implications: a review." *J Am Coll Nutr,* vol. 13, no. 5, pp. 429–446, 1994

17. Blaylock RL, *Excitotoxins: The Taste That Kills,* Health Press, Sante Fe, NM, 1997

18. Ibid.

19. Seelig MS, "Athletic stress, performance and magnesium in consequences of magnesium deficiency on the enhancement of stress reactions; preventive and therapeutic implications: a review." *J Am Coll Nutr,* vol. 13, no. 5, pp. 429–446, 1994

20. Singh RB, "Effect of dietary magnesium supplementation in the prevention of coronary heart disease and sudden cardiac death." *Magnesium Trace Elem,* vol. 9, pp. 143–151, 1990

21. Stendig–Lindberg G, "Sudden death of athletes: is it due to long-term changes in serum magnesium, lipids and blood sugar?" *J Basic Clin Physiol Pharmacol,* vol. 3, no. 2, pp. 153–164, 1992

CHAPTER 4

1. Blaylock RL, *Excitotoxins: The Taste That Kills,* Health Press, Sante Fe, NM, 1997

2. Ibid.

3. Eades M, Eades A, *The Protein Power Lifeplan,* Warner Books, New York, 1999

4. Seelig MS, "Review and hypothesis: might patients with chronic fatigue syndrome have latent tetany of magnesium deficiency." *J Chron Fatigue Syndr,* vol. 4, no. 2, pp. 77–108, 1998

5. Weaver K, "Magnesium and migraine." *Headache,* vol. 30, p. 168, 1990

6. Mauskop A, Fox B, *What Your Doctor May Not Tell You About Migraines,* Warner Books, New York, 2001

7. Mauskop A et al., "Deficiency in serum ionized magnesium but not total magnesium in patients with migraines. Possible role of ICa2+/IMg2+ ratio." *Headache,* vol. 33, no. 3, pp. 135–138, 1993

8. Mauskop A et al., "Intravenous magnesium sulphate relieves migraine attacks in patients with low serum ionized magnesium levels: a pilot study." *Clin Sci (Colch),* vol. 89, no. 6, pp. 633–636, 1995

9. Mauskop A, Altura BT et al., "Intravenous magnesium sulfate rapidly alleviates headaches of various types." *Headache,* vol. 36, no. 3, pp. 154–160, 1996

10. Mauskop A, Altura BM, "Role of magnesium in the pathogenesis and treatment of migraines." *Clin Neurosci,* vol. 83, no. 5, pp. 24–27, 1998

11. Mauskop A et al., "Intravenous magnesium sulfate relieves cluster headaches in patients with low serum ionized magnesium levels." *Headache,* vol. 35, no. 10, pp. 597–600, 1995

12. Mauskop A, Altura BT et al., "Intravenous magnesium sulfate rapidly alleviates headaches of various types." *Headache,* vol. 36, no. 3, pp. 154–160, 1996

13. Peikert A, Wilimzig C et al., "Prophylaxis of migraine with oral magnesium: results from a prospective, multi-center, placebo-controlled and double-blind randomized study." *Cephalalgia,* vol. 16, no. 4, pp. 257–263, 1996

14. Institute of Medicine, *Dietary Reference Intake for Calcium, Phosphorus, Magnesium, Vitamin D, and Fluoride,* National Academy Press, Washington DC, 1997

15. Blaylock RL, *Excitotoxins: The Taste That Kills,* Health Press, Sante Fe, NM, 1997

16. Durlach J et al., "Physiopathology of symptomatic and latent forms of central nervous hyperexcitability due to magnesium deficiency: a current general scheme." *Magnes Res,* vol. 13, no. 4, pp. 293–302, 2000

17. Cernak I et al., "Characterization of plasma magnesium concentration and oxidative stress following graded traumatic brain injury in humans." *J Neurotrauma,* vol. 17, no. 1, pp. 53–68, 2000

18. Memon ZI et al., "Predictive value of serum ionized but not total magnesium levels in head injuries." *Scand J Clin Lab Invest,* vol. 55, no. 8, pp. 671–677, 1995

19. Heath DL, Vink R, "Brain free magnesium concentration is predictive of motor outcome following traumatic axonal brain injury in rats." *Magnes Res,* vol. 12, no. 4, pp. 269–277, 1999

20. Blaylock, ibid.

21. Marcus JC et al., "Serum ionized magnesium in post-traumatic headaches." *J Pediatr,* vol. 139, no. 3, pp. 459–462, 2001

22. Altura BM, Altura BT, "Association of alcohol in brain injury, headaches, and stroke with brain-tissue and serum levels of ionized magnesium: a review of recent findings and mechanisms of action." *Alcohol,* vol. 19, no. 2, pp. 119–130, 1999

23. Altura BM et al., "Alcohol-induced spasms of cerebral blood vessels: relation to cerebrovascular accidents and sudden death." *Science,* vol. 220, no. 4594, pp. 331–333, 1983

24. Zhang A et al., "Chronic treatment of cultured cerebral vascular smooth cells with low concentration of ethanol elevates intracellular calcium and potentiates prostanoid-induced rises in [Ca2+]i: relation to etiology of alcohol-induced stroke." *Alcohol,* vol. 14, no. 4, pp. 367–371, 1997

25. Altura BM, Altura BT, "Association of alcohol in brain injury, headaches, and stroke with brain-tissue and serum levels of ionized magnesium: a review of recent findings and mechanisms of action." *Alcohol,* vol. 19, no. 2, pp. 119–130, 1999

26. Ibid.

27. Altura BM et al., "Extracellular magnesium regulates nuclear and perinuclear free ionized calcium in cerebral vascular smooth muscle cells: possible relation to alcohol and central nervous system injury." *Alcohol,* vol. 23, no. 2, pp. 83–90, 2001

28. Ema M et al., "Alcohol-induced vascular damage of brain is ameliorated by administration of magnesium." *Alcohol,* vol. 15, no. 2, pp. 95–103, 1998

29. Altura BM, Altura BT, "Association of alcohol in brain injury, headaches, and stroke with brain-tissue and serum levels of ionized magnesium: a review of recent findings and mechanisms of action." *Alcohol,* vol. 19, no. 2, pp. 119–130, 1999

30. Li W et al., "Antioxidants prevent depletion of [Mg2+]i induced by alcohol in cultured canine cerebral vascular smooth muscle cells: possible relationship to alcohol-induced stroke." *Brain Res Bull,* vol. 55, no. 4, pp. 475–478, 2001

31. Horn B, "Magnesium and the cardiovascular system." *Magnesium,* vol. 6, pp. 109–111, 1987

32. Schulz-Stubner S et al., "Magnesium as part of balanced general anaesthesia with propofol, remifentanil and mivacurium: a double-blind, randomized prospective study in 50 patients." *Eur J Anaesthesiol,* vol. 18, no. 11, pp. 723–729, 2001

33. Yang CY, "Calcium and magnesium in drinking water and risk of death from cerebrovascular disease." *Stroke,* vol. 18, no. 8, pp. 411–414, 1998

34. Altura BT, Altura BM, "Withdrawal of magnesium causes vasospasm while elevated magnesium produces relaxation of tone in cerebral arteries." *Neurosci Lett,* vol. 20, no. 3, pp. 323–327, 1980

35. Altura BT, Altura BM, "Interactions of Mg and K on cerebral vessels—aspects in view of stroke. Review of present status and new findings." *Magnesium,* vol. 3, nos. 4–6, pp. 195–211, 1984

36. Li W et al., "Antioxidants prevent elevation in [Ca(2+)](i) induced by low extracellular magnesium in cultured canine cerebral vascular smooth muscle cells: possible relationship to Mg(2+) deficiency-induced vasospasm and stroke." *Brain Res Bull,* vol. 52, no. 2, pp. 151–154, 2000

37. Blaylock RL, *Excitotoxins: The Taste That Kills,* Health Press, Sante Fe, NM, 1997

38. Ibid.

39. Altura BT et al., "Low levels of serum ionized magnesium are found in patients early after stroke which result in rapid elevation in cytosolic free calcium and spasm in cerebral vascular muscle cells." *Neurosci Lett,* vol. 230, no. 1, pp. 37–40, 1997

40. Rothman SM, Olney JW, "Glutamate and the pathophysiology of hypoxic-ischemic brain damage." *Ann Neurol,* vol. 19, pp. 105–111, 1986

41. Galland L, *Superimmunity for Kids,* Bantam Doubleday Dell, New York, 1988

CHAPTER 5

1. Goldberg B, *Heart Disease,* Future Medicine Publication, Tiburon, CA, 1998

2. Sei M et al., "Nutritional epidemiological study on mineral intake and mortality from cardiovascular disease. Tokushima." *J Exp Med,* vol. 40, pp. 199–207, 1993

3. Zwillinger L, "Effect of magnesium on the heart." *Klin Wochenschr,* vol. 14, pp. 1429–1433, 1935

4. Tom Miller, personal communication, March 2001.

5. Singh RB, "Magnesium status and risk of coronary artery disease in rural and urban populations with variable magnesium consumption." *Magnes Res,* vol. 10, no. 3, pp. 205–213, 1997

6. Liao F, Folsom AR, "Is low magnesium concentration a risk factor for coronary heart disease? The atherosclerosis risk in communities (ARIC) study." *Am Heart J,* vol. 136, no. 3, pp. 480–490, 1998

7. Ford, Earl S. "Serum magnesium and ischemic heart disease: findings from a national sample of US adults." *International Journal of Epidemiology,* vol. 28, pp. 645–651, 1999

8. Seelig MS et al., "Magnesium interrelationships in ischemic heart disease: a review." *American Journal of Clinical Nutrition,* Jan. 1974

9. Sherer Y, Bitzur R, Cohen H, Shaish A, Varon D, Shoenfeld Y, Harats D, "Mechanisms of action of the anti-atherogenic effect of magnesium: lessons from a mouse model." *Magnes Res,* vol. 14, no. 3, pp. 173–179, 2001

10. Morrill GA, Gupta RK, Kostellow AB, Ma GY, Zhang A, Altura BT, Altura BM, "Mg2+ modulates membrane sphingolipid and lipid second messenger levels in vascular smooth muscle cells." *FEBS Lett,* vol. 440, nos. 1–2, pp. 167–171, 1998

11. Yang ZW, Gebrewold A et al., "Mg++-induced endothelial-dependent relaxation of blood vessels and blood pressure lowering: role of NO." *Am J Physiol Regul Integr Comp Physiol.* vol. 278, pp. R628–639, 2000

12. Goldberg B, *Heart Disease,* Future Medicine Publication, Tiburon, CA, 1998

13. Altura BT et al., "Magnesium dietary intake modulates blood lipid levels and arherogenesis." *Proc Natl Acad Sci,* vol. 87, no. 5, pp. 1840–1844, 1990

14. Singh RB et al., "Does dietary magnesium modulate blood lipids?" *Biol Trace Elem Res,* vol. 30, pp. 50–64, 1991

15. Corica F et al., "Effects of oral magnesium supplementation on plasma lipid concentrations in patients with non-insulin-dependent diabetes mellitus." *Magnesium Res,* vol. 7, pp. 43–46, 1994

16. Durlach J, "Commentary on recent epidemiological and clinical advances." *Magnesium Research,* vol. 9, no. 2, pp. 139–141, 1996

17. Fallon S, Enig M, *Nourishing Traditions,* Locomotion Press, Baltimore, MD, 1995

18. Gao M et al., "Cardiovascular risk factors emerging in Chinese populations undergoing urbanization." *Hypertens Res,* vol. 22, pp. 209–215, 1999

19. Marier JR, "Magnesium content of the food supply in the modern-day world." *Magnesium,* vol. 5, pp. 1–8, 1986

20. Liu L et al., "Comparative studies of diet-related factors and blood pressure among Chinese and Japanese: results from the China-Japan Cooperative Research of the WHO-CARDIAC Study. Cardiovascular disease and alimentary comparison." *Hypertens Res,* vol. 23, pp. 413–420, 2000

21. McCully KS, "Homocysteine, folate, vitamin B_6, and cardiovascular disease." *JAMA,* vol. 279, no. 5, pp. 392–393, 1998

22. McCully KS, "Vascular pathology of homocysteinemia: implications for the pathogenesis of arteriosclerosis." *Am J Pathol,* vol. 56, no. 1, pp. 111–128, 1969

23. Eikelboom JW et al., "Preventive cardiology and therapeutics program." *Ann Intern Med,* vol. 131, no. 5, pp. 363–375, 1999

24. Boushey CJ et al., "A quantitative assessment of plasma homocysteine as a risk factor for vascular disease. Probable benefits of increasing folic acid intakes." *JAMA,* vol. 274, no. 13, pp. 1049–1057, 1995

25. Confalonieri M et al., "Heterozygosity for homocysteinuria: a detectable and reversible risk factor for pulmonary thromboembolism." *Monaldi Arch Chest Disease,* vol. 50, no. 2, pp. 114–115, 1995

26. Altura B, Altura B, "Magnesium: the forgotten mineral in cardiovascular health and disease." A Gem Lecture at SUNY Downstate. *Alumni Today,* pp. 11–22, spring 2001

27. Li W et al., "Extracellular magnesium regulates effects of vitamin B_6, B_{12} and folate on homocysteinemia-induced depletion of intracellular free magnesium ions in canine cerebral vascular smooth muscle cells: possible relationship to [Ca2+]i, atherogenesis and stroke." *Neurosci Lett,* vol. 274, no. 2, pp. 83–86, 1999

28. Shamsuddin AM, "Inositol phosphates have novel anti-cancer function." *Journal of Nutrition,* vol. 125 (suppl.), pp. 725S–732S, Review 1995

29. Rowley KG et al., "Improvements in circulating cholesterol, anti-oxidants, and homocysteine after dietary intervention in an Australian Aboriginal community." *Am J Clin Nutr,* vol. 74, no. 4, pp. 442–448, 2001

30. Tice JA et al., "Cost-effectiveness of vitamin therapy to lower plasma homocysteine levels for the prevention of coronary heart disease: effect of grain fortification and beyond." *JAMA,* vol. 286, no. 8, pp. 936–943, 2001

31. Vollset SE et al., "Plasma total homocysteine and cardiovascular and noncardiovascular mortality: the Hordaland Homocysteine Study." *Am J Clin Nutr,* vol. 74, no. 1, pp. 130–136, 2001

32. *Physicians' Desk Reference*

33. Altura BM et al., "Hypomagnesemia and vasoconstriction: possible relationship to etiology of sudden death ischemic heart disease and hypertensive vascular diseases." *Artery,* vol. 9, no. 3, pp. 212–231, 1981

34. Mindell E, *Prescription Alternatives,* Keats Publishing, Los Angeles, 1999

35. Millane T, Camm A, *Medical Sciences Bulletin,* Pharmaceutical Information Associates, May 1994

36. Kisters K et al., "Hypomagnesaemia, borderline hypertension and hyperlipidaemia." *Magnesium Bull,* vol. 21, pp. 31–34, 1999

37. Altura BM, Altura BT et al., "Magnesium deficiency and hypertension: correlation between magnesium-deficient diets and microcirculatory changes in situ." *Science,* vol. 223, no. 4642, pp. 1315–1317, 1984

38. Resnick LM et al., "Factors affecting blood pressure responses to diet: the Vanguard study." *Am J Hypertens,* vol. 13, no. 9, pp. 956–965, 2000

39. Altura BM, Altura BT, "Interactions of Mg and K on blood vessels—aspects in view of hypertension. Review of present status and new findings." *Magnesium,* vol. 3, nos. 4–6, pp. 175–194, 1984

40. Pierce JB, *Heart Healthy Magnesium: Your Nutritional Key to Cardiovascular Wellness,* Avery Publishing Group, New York, 1994

41. Shechter M et al., "Beneficial antithrombotic effects of the association of pharmacological oral magnesium therapy with aspirin in coronary heart disease patients." *Magnes Research,* vol. 13, no. 4, pp. 275–284, 2000

42. Zwillinger L, "Effect of magnesium on the heart." *Klin Wochenschr,* vol. 14, pp. 1429–1433, 1935

43. Boyd LJ et al., "Magnesium sulfate in paroxysmal tachycardia." *Am J Med Sci,* vol. 206, pp. 43–48, 1943

44. Teo KK et al., "Effects of intravenous magnesium in suspected acute myocardial infarction: Overview of randomized trials." *Brit Med J,* vol. 303, pp. 1499–1503, 1991

45. Teo KK, Yusuf S, "Role of magnesium in reducing mortality in acute myocardial infarction. A review of the evidence." *Drugs,* vol. 46, pp. 347–359, 1993

46. Woods KL et al., "Intravenous magnesium sulfate in suspected acute myocardial infarction: results of the second Leicester Intravenous Magnesium Intervention Trial (LIMIT-2)." *Lancet,* vol. 339, pp. 1553–1558, 1992.

47. Woods KL, Fletcher S, "Long-term outcome after intravenous magnesium sulphate in suspected acute myocardial infarction: the second Leicester Intravenous Magnesium Intervention Trial (LIMIT-2)," *Lancet,* vol. 343, pp. 816–819, 1994

48. Ravn HB, "Pharmacological effects of magnesium on arterial thrombosis—mechanisms of action?" *Magnes Research,* vol. 12, no. 3, pp. 191–199, 1999

49. Young IS et al., "Magnesium status and digoxin toxicity." *Br J Clin Pharmacol,* vol. 32, no. 6, pp. 717–721, 1991

50. Lewis R et al., "Magnesium deficiency may be an important determinant of ventricular ectopy in digitalised patients with chronic atrial fibrillation." *Br J Clin Pharmacol,* vol. 31, no. 2, pp. 200–203, 1991

51. ISIS-4 (Fourth International Study of Infarct Survival) Collaborative Group, "ISIS-4: a randomised factorial trial assessing early oral captopril, oral mononitrate, and intravenous magnesium sulphate in 58,050 patients with suspected acute myocardial infarction." *Lancet,* vol. 345, pp. 669–685, 1995

52. Seelig MS, "Cardiovascular reactions to stress intensified by magnesium deficit in consequences of magnesium deficiency on the enhancement of stress reactions; preventive and therapeutic implications: a review." *J Am Coll Nutr,* vol. 13, no. 5, pp. 429–446, 1994

53. Shechter M et al., "Magnesium therapy in acute myocardial infarc-

tion when patients are not cardiologists for thrombolytic therapy." *AM J Cardiology,* vol. 75, pp. 321–323, 1995.

54. Pierce JB, *Heart Healthy Magnesium: Your Nutritional Key to Cardiovascular Wellness,* Avery Publishing Group, New York, 1994

55. Iseri LT, "Magnesium and cardiac arrhythmias." *Magnesium,* vol. 5, nos. 3–4, pp. 111–126, 1986

56. Iseri LT, Allen BJ, "Magnesium therapy of cardiac arrhythmias in critical-care medicine." *Magnesium,* vol. 8, pp. 299–306, 1989

57. Perticone F et al., "Antiarrhythmic short-term protective magnesium treatment in ischemic dilated cardiomyopathy." *J Am Coll Nutr,* vol. 5, no. 3, pp. 492–499, 1990

58. Pierce JB, *Heart Healthy Magnesium: Your Nutritional Key to Cardiovascular Wellness,* Avery Publishing Group, New York, 1994

59. Boyd LJ et al., "Magnesium sulfate in paroxysmal tachycardia." *Am J Med Sci,* vol. 206, pp. 43–48, 1943

60. Parikka HJ, Toivonen LK, "Acute effects of intravenous magnesium on ventricular refractoriness and monophasic action potential duration in humans." *Scand Cardiovasc J,* vol. 33, no. 5, pp. 300–305, 1999

61. Thiele R, Protze F, Winnefeld K, Pfeifer R, Pleissner J, Gassel M, "Effect of intravenous magnesium on ventricular tachyarrhythmias associated with acute myocardial infarction." *Magnes Res,* vol. 13, no. 2, pp. 111–112, 2000

62. Ceremuzynski L et al., "Hypomagnesaemia in heart failure with ventricular arrhythmias. Beneficial effects of magnesium supplementation." *J Intern Med,* vol. 247, pp. 78–86, 2000

63. Dyckner T et al., "Magnesium deficiency in congestive heart failure." *Acta Pharmacol Toxicol Copenh,* vol. 54, suppl. 1, pp. 119–123, 1984

64. England MR et al., "Magnesium administration and dysrhythmias after cardiac surgery." *JAMA,* vol. 268, pp. 2395–2402, 1992

65. Caspi J et al., "Effects of magnesium on myocardial function after coronary artery bypass grafting." *Ann Thorac Surg,* vol. 59, pp. 942–947, 1995

66. Toraman F, Karabulut EH, Alhan HC, Dagdelen S, Tarcan S, "Magnesium infusion dramatically decreases the incidence of atrial fibrillation after coronary artery bypass grafting." *Ann Thorac Surg,* vol. 72, no. 4, pp. 1256–1261, 2001

67. Seelig MS, "Review and hypothesis: might patients with the chronic fatigue syndrome have latent tetany of magnesium deficiency." *J Chron Fatigue Syndr,* vol. 4, pp. 77–108, 1998

68. Lichodziejewsa B et al., "Clinical symptoms of mitral valve prolapse are related to hypomagnesemia and attenuated by magnesium supplementation." *Amer J Cardiology,* vol. 79, pp. 768–772, 1997

CHAPTER 6

1. Singh RB, "Association of low plasma concentrations of antioxidant vitamins, magnesium and zinc with high body fat per cent in Indian men." *Magnes Res,* vol. 11, no. 1, pp. 3–10, 1998

2. Ma J et al., "Associations of serum and dietary magnesium with cardiovascular disease, hypertension, diabetes, insulin, and carotid arterial wall thickness; the ARIC study, Artherosclerosis Risk in Communities Study." *J Clin Epidemiol,* vol. 48, pp. 927–940, 1995

3. Humphries S et al., "Low dietary magnesium is associated with insulin resistance in a sample of young, non-diabetic Black Americans." *Am J Hypertens,* vol. 12, no. 8, pt. 1, pp. 747–756, 1999

4. Alzaid AA et al., "Effects of insulin on plasma magnesium in noninsulin-dependent diabetes mellitus: evidence for insulin resistance." *J Clin Endocrinol Metab,* vol. 80, no. 4, pp. 1376–1381, 1995

5. Barbagallo M et al., "Altered cellular magnesium responsiveness to hyperglycemia in hypertensive subjects." *Hypertension,* vol. 38, no. 3 pt. 2, pp. 612–615, 2001

6. Dominguez LJ et al., "Magnesium responsiveness to insulin and insulin-like growth factor I in erythrocytes from normotensive and hypertensive subjects." *J Clin Endocrinol Metab,* vol. 83, no. 12, pp. 4402–4407, 1998

7. Resnick LM, "Cellular ions in hypertension, insulin resistance, obesity, and diabetes: a unifying theme." *J Am Soc Nephrol,* vol. 3 (4 suppl.), pp. 578–585, 1992

8. Karppanen H, Neuvonen PJ, "Ischaemic heart-disease and soil magnesium in Finland: water hardness and magnesium in heart muscle." *The Lancet,* Dec. 15, 1973

9. Resnick LM, "Ionic basis of hypertension, insulin resistance, vascular disease, and related disorders. The mechanism of syndrome X." *Am J Hypertens,* vol. 6, no. 5, pt. 1, pp. 413–417, 1993

10. Resnick LM, "The cellular ionic basis of hypertension and allied clinical conditions." *Prog Cardiovasc Dis,* vol. 42, pp. 1–22, 1999

11. Resnick LM et al., "Hypertension and peripheral insulin resistance. Possible mediating role of intracellular free magnesium." *Am J Hypertens,* vol. 3, no. 5, pt. 1, pp. 373–379, 1990

12. Paolisso G et al., "Low fasting and insulin-mediated intracellular magnesium accumulation in hypertensive patients with left ventricular hypertrophy; role of insulin resistance." *Hypertens,* vol. 9, pp. 199–203, 1995

13. Nadler JL et al., "Magnesium deficiency produces insulin resistance and increased thromboxane synthesis." *Hypertension,* vol. 21, no. 6, pt. 2, pp. 1024–1029, 1993

14. Bardicef M et al., "Extracellular and intracellular magnesium depletion in pregnancy and gestational diabetes." *Am J Obstet Gynecol,* vol. 172, no. 3, pp. 1009–1013, 1995

15. Resnick LM et al., "Intracellular and extracellular magnesium depletion in type 2 (non-insulin-dependent) diabetes mellitus." *Diabetologia,* vol. 36, no. 8, pp. 767–770, 1993

16. Kao WH et al., "Serum and dietary magnesium and the risk for type 2 diabetes mellitus: the Atherosclerosis Risk in Communities Study." *Arch Intern Med,* vol. 159, no. 18, pp. 2151–2159, 1999

17. Lima M de L, "The effect of magnesium supplementation in increasing doses on the control of type 2 diabetes." *Diabetes Care,* vol. 83, no. 5, pp. 682–686, 1998

18. Paolisso G, Barbagallo M, "Hypertension, diabetes mellitus, and insulin resistance: the role of intracellular magnesium." *Am J Hypertens,* vol. 10, no. 3, pp. 346–355, 1997

19. Merz CN et al., "Oral magnesium supplementation inhibits platelet-dependent thrombosis in patients with coronary artery disease." *Am J Cardiol,* vol. 84, pp. 152–156, 1999

20. Lima M de L, "The effect of magnesium supplementation in increasing doses on the control of type 2 diabetes." *Diabetes Care,* vol. 83, no. 5, pp. 682–686, 1998

21. Engelen W, Bouten A, De Leeuw I, De Block C, "Are low magnesium levels in type 1 diabetes associated with electromyographical signs of polyneuropathy?" *Magnes Res,* vol. 13, no. 3, pp. 197–203, 2000

22. Djurhuus MS et al., "Effect of moderate improvement in metabolic control on magnesium and lipid concentrations in patients with type 1 diabetes." *Diabetes Care,* vol. 22, no. 4, pp. 546–554, 1999

23. Squires S, "The amazing statistics and dangers of soda pop." *Washington Post,* February 27, 2001, p. HE10.

24. Ludwig DS et al., "Relation between consumption of sugar-sweetened drinks and childhood obesity: a prospective, observational analysis." *Lancet,* vol. 357, no. 9255, pp. 505–508, 2001

25. Bernstein J et al., "Depression of lymphocyte transformation following oral glucose ingestion." *Am J Clin Nutr,* vol. 30, p. 613, 1977

26. Sanchez A et al., "Role of sugars in human neutrophilic phagocytosis." *Am J Clin Nutr,* vol. 26, no. 11, pp. 1180–1184, 1973

27. Kijak E et al., "Relationship of blood sugar level and leukocytic phagocytosis." *S Calif State Dent Assoc J,* vol. 32, no. 9, 1964

28. Lima M de L, "The effect of magnesium supplementation in increasing doses on the control of type 2 diabetes." *Diabetes Care,* vol. 83, no. 5, pp. 682–686, 1998

29. Yang CY et al., "Magnesium in drinking water and the risk of death from diabetes mellitus." *Magnes Res,* vol. 12, no. 2, pp. 131–137, 1999

30. Zhao HX et al., "Drinking water composition and childhood-onset type 1 diabetes mellitus in Devon and Cornwall, England." *Diabet Med,* vol. 18, no. 9, pp. 709–717, 2001

31. Howard JMH, "Magnesium deficiency in peripheral vascular disease." *J Nutritional Med,* vol. 1, p. 39, 1990

32. Roberts HJ, *Aspartame Disease: An Ignored Epidemic.* Sunshine Sentinel Press, West Palm Beach, FL, 2001

CHAPTER 7

1. Werbach M, "Premenstrual syndrome: magnesium." *Townsend Letter for Doctors,* June 1995, p. 26

2. Sherwood RA et al., "Magnesium and the premenstrual syndrome." *Ann. Clin. Biochem,* vol. 23, no. 6, pp. 667–670, 1986

3. Posaci et al., "Plasma copper, zinc and magnesium levels in patients with premenstrual tension syndrome." *ACTA Obstetrics and Gynecology Scand,* vol. 73, no. 6, pp. 452–455, 1994

4. Facchinetti F et al., "Oral magnesium successfully relieves premen-

strual mood changes." *Obstetrics and Gynecology (USA)*, vol. 78, no. 2, pp. 177–181, 1991

5. Somer E, *The Essential Guide to Vitamins and Minerals*, Harper-Collins, New York 1995

6. Murray M, *Encyclopedia of Natural Medicine*, 2nd ed, Prima Publishing, Rocklin, CA, 1998

7. Muneyvirci-Delale O et al., "Sex steroid hormones modulate serum ionized magnesium and calcium levels throughout the menstrual cycle in women." *Fertil Steril*, vol. 69, no. 5, pp. 58–62, 1998

8. Li W et al., "Sex steroid hormones exert biphasic effects on cytosolic magnesium ions in cerebral vascular smooth muscle cells: possible relationships to migraine frequency in premenstrual syndromes and stroke incidence." *Brain Res Bull*, vol. 54, no. 1, pp. 83–89, 2001

9. Marz R, *Medical Nutrition from Marz*, 2nd ed. Omni Press, Portland, OR, 1997

10. Benassi L et al., "Effectiveness of magnesium pidolate in the prophylactic treatment of primary dysmenorrhea." *Clin Exp Obstet Gynecol*, vol. 19, no. 3, pp. 176–179, 1992

11. Fontana-Klaiber H, Hogg B, "Therapeutic effects of magnesium in dysmenorrhea." *Schweiz Rundsch Med Prax*, vol. 79, no. 16, pp. 491–494, 1990

12. Seifert B et al., "Magnesium—a new therapeutic alternative in primary dysmenorrhea." *Zentralbl Gynakol*, vol. 111, no. 11, pp. 755–760, 1989

13. Goldberg B, *Alternative Medicine Guide: Women's Health Series 1*, Future Medicine Publication, Tiburon, CA, 1998

14. Franz KB, "Magnesium intake during pregnancy." *Magnesium*, vol. 6, pp. 18–27, 1987

15. Muneyvirci-Delale O et al., "Divalent cations in women with PCOS: implications for cardiovascular disease." *Gynecol Endocrinol*, vol. 15, no. 3, pp. 198–201, 2001

16. Conradt A, Weidinger AH, "The central position of magnesium in the management of fetal hypotrophy—a contribution to the pathomechanism of utero-placental insufficiency, prematurity and poor intrauterine fetal growth as well as pre-eclampsia." *Magnesium Bull*, vol. 4, pp. 103–124, 1982

17. Handwerker SM et al., "Ionized serum magnesium levels in

umbilical cord blood of normal pregnant women at delivery: relationship to calcium, demographics, and birthweight." *Am J Perinatol,* vol. 10, no. 5, pp. 392–397, 1993

18. Handwerker SM, Altura BT, Altura BM, "Serum ionized magnesium and other electrolytes in the antenatal period of human pregnancy." *J Am Coll Nutr,* vol. 15, no. 1, pp. 36–43, 1996

19. Lazard EM, "A preliminary report on the intravenous use of magnesium sulphate in puerperal eclampsia." *Am J Obst Gynec,* vol. 9, pp. 178–188, 1925

20. Seelig MS, *Magnesium Deficiency in the Pathogenesis of Disease. Early Roots of Cardiovascular, Skeletal, and Renal Abnormalities,* Plenum, New York, 1980

21. Almonte RA et al., "Gestational magnesium deficiency is deleterious to fetal outcome." *Biol Neonate,* vol. 76, no. 1, pp. 26–32, 1999

22. Seelig MS, "Toxemias of pregnancy, postpartum cardiomyopathy and SIDS in consequences of magnesium deficiency on the enhancement of stress reactions; preventive and therapeutic implications: a review." *J Am Coll Nutr,* vol. 13, no. 5, pp. 429–446, 1994

23. Seelig MS, "Prenatal and neonatal mineral deficiencies: magnesium, zinc and chromium." In *Clinical Disorders in Pediatric Nutrition,* Marcel Dekker, New York, pp. 167–196, 1982

24. Seelig MS, "Magnesium in pregnancy: special needs for the adolescent mother." *J Am Coll Nutr,* vol. 10, p. 566, 1991

25. Caddell JL, "Magnesium deficiency promotes muscle weakness, contributing to the risk of sudden infant death (SIDS) in infants sleeping prone." *Magnes Res,* vol. 14, nos. 1–2, pp. 39–50, 2001

26. Caddell JL, "A triple-risk model for the sudden infant death syndrome (SIDS) and the apparent life-threatening episode (ALTE): the stressed magnesium deficient weanling rat." *Magnes Res,* vol. 14, no. 3, pp. 227–238, 2001

27. Durlach J et al., "Magnesium and thermoregulation. I. Newborn and infant. Is sudden infant death syndrome a magnesium-dependent disease of the transition from chemical to physical thermoregulation." *Magnes Res,* vol. 4, pp. 137–152, 1991

28. Nelson KB et al., "Can magnesium sulfate reduce the risk of cerebral palsy in very low birth weight infants?" *Pediatrics,* vol. 95, no. 2, 1995

29. Schendel D et al., "Prenatal magnesium sulfate exposure and the risk

for cerebral palsy or mental retardation among very low birth-weight children aged 3–5 years." *JAMA,* vol. 276, pp. 1805–1810, 1996

30. Dedhia HV, Banks DE, "Pulmonary response to hyperoxia: effects of magnesium." *Environ Health Perspect,* vol. 102, suppl. 10, pp. 101–105, 1994

31. Oorschot DE, "Cerebral palsy and experimental hypoxia-induced perinatal brain injury: is magnesium protective?" *Magnes Res,* vol. 13, no. 4, pp. 265–273, 2000

32. Bara M, Guiet-Bara A, "Magnesium regulation of Ca2+ channels in smooth muscle and endothelial cells of human allantochorial placental vessels." *Magnes Research,* vol. 14, nos. 1–2, pp. 11–18, 2001

CHAPTER 8

1. Brown S, *Better Bones, Better Body,* Keats Publishing, New Canaan, CT, 1996

2. Thomas AJ et al., "Ca, Mg and P status of elderly inpatients: dietary intake, metabolic balance studies and biochemical status." *Br. J. Nutr,* vol. 62, pp. 211–219, 1989

3. Bunker VW, "Osteoporosis in the elderly." *Br J Biomed Sci,* vol. 51, no. 3, pp. 228–240, 1994

4. The National Institutes of Health Osteoporosis Prevention, Diagnosis, and Therapy Consensus Statement, Mar. 2000

5. Rude RK, "Magnesium deficiency-induced osteoporosis in the rat: uncoupling of bone formation and bone resorption." *Magnes Research,* vol. 12, no. 4, pp. 257–267, 1999

6. Rude RK et al., "Magnesium deficiency induces bone loss in the rat." *Miner Electrolyte Metab,* vol. 24, no. 5, pp. 314–320, 1998

7. Brodowski J, "Levels of ionized magnesium in women with various stages of postmenopausal osteoporosis progression evaluated on the basis of densitometric examinations." *Przegl Lek,* vol. 57, no. 12, pp. 714–716, 2000

8. Sojka JE, Weaver CM, "Magnesium supplementation and osteoporosis." *Nutrition Reviews,* vol. 53, p. 71, 1995.

9. Goldberg B, *Alternative Medicine Guide: Women's Health Series 2,* Future Medicine Publishing, Tiburon, CA, 1998

10. Dreosti IE, "Magnesium status and health." *Nutrition Reviews,* vol. 53, no. 9, pp. 523–527, 1995

11. Abraham GE, Grewal HA, "Total dietary program emphasizing magnesium instead of calcium: effect on the mineral density of calcaneous bone in postmenopausal women on hormonal therapy." *Journal of Reproductive Medicine,* vol. 35, no. 5, pp. 503–507, 1990

12. Seelig MS, "Increased magnesium need with use of combined estrogen and calcium for osteoporosis." *Magnesium Res,* vol. 3, pp. 197–215, 1990

13. Goldberg B, *Alternative Medicine Guide: Women's Health Series 2,* Future Medicine Publishing, Tiburon, CA, 1998

14. Brown S, *Better Bones, Better Body,* Keats Publishing, New Canaan, CT, 1996

15. Tucker KL et al., "Potassium, magnesium, and fruit and vegetable intakes are associated with greater bone mineral density in elderly men and women." *Am J Clin Nutr,* vol. 69, no. 4, pp. 727–736, 1999

16. Hall WD et al., "Risk factors for kidney stones in older women in the southern United States." *Am J Med Sci,* vol. 322, no. 1, pp. 12–18, 2001

17. Milne DB, Nielsen FH, "The interaction between dietary fructose and magnesium adversely affects macromineral homeostasis in men." *J Am Coll Nutr,* vol. 19, no. 1, pp. 31–37, 2000

18. Institute of Medicine. *Dietary Reference Intake for Calcium, Phosphorus, Magnesium, Vitamin D, and Fluoride,* National Academy Press, Washington DC, 1997

19. Milne D, Nielsen F, "Too much soda may take some fizz out of the bones." *Proc ND Acad Sci,* vol. 51, p. 212, 1998

20. Bunce GE et al., "Distribution of calcium and magnesium in rat kidney homogenate fractions accompanying magnesium deficiency induced nephrocalcinosis." *Exp Mol Pathol,* vol. 21, no. 1, pp. 16–28, 1974

21. Johansson G et al., "Effects of magnesium hydroxide in renal stone disease." *J Am Coll Nutr,* vol. 1, no. 2, 1982

22. Prien EL, "Magnesium oxide-pyridoxine therapy for recurring calcium oxalate urinary calculi." *J Urology,* vol. 112, pp. 509–551, 1974

23. Johannson G et al., "Biochemical and clinical effects of prophylactic treatment of renal calcium stones with magnesium hydroxide." *J Urol,* vol. 124, pp. 770–774, 1980

24. Driessens FC, Verbeeck RM, "On the prevention and treatment of cal-

cification disorders of old age." *Med Hypotheses,* vol. 3, pp. 131–137, 1988

25. Labeeuw M et al., "Role of magnesium in the physiopathology and treatment of calcium renal lithiasis." *Presse Med,* vol. 16, no. 1, pp. 25–27, 1987

26. Jeppesen BB, "Greenland, a soft-water area with a low incidence of ischemic heart death." *Magnesium,* vol. 6, no. 6, pp. 307–313, 1987

CHAPTER 9

1. Goldstein JA, ed., *Chronic Fatigue Syndromes: The Limbic Hypothesis,* Haworth Press, New York, 1993

2. Seelig MS, "Review and hypothesis: might patients with the chronic fatigue syndrome have latent tetany of magnesium deficiency." *J Chron Fatigue Syndr,* vol. 4, pp. 77–108, 1998

3. Papadopol V, Tuchendria E, Palamaru I, "Magnesium and some psychological features in two groups of pupils (magnesium and psychic features)." *Magnes Research,* vol. 14, nos. 1–2, pp. 27–32, 2001

4. Durlach V et al., "Neurotic, neuromuscular and autonomic nervous form of magnesium imbalance." *Magnes Res,* vol. 10, pp. 169–195, 1997

5. Cox IM, "Red blood cell magnesium and chronic fatigue syndrome." *The Lancet,* vol. 337, pp. 757–760, 1991

6. Goldberg B, *Chronic Fatigue, Fibromyalgia & Environmental Illness: 26 Doctors Show You How They Reverse These Conditions with Clinically Proven Alternative Therapies,* Future Medicine Publishing, Tiburon, CA, 1998

7. Ibid.

8. Seelig MS, "Athletic stress, performance and magnesium in consequences of magnesium deficiency on the enhancement of stress reactions; preventive and therapeutic implications: a review" *J Am Coll Nutr,* vol. 13, no. 5, pp. 429–446, 1994

9. Abraham GE, Flechas JD, "Management of fibromyalgia: rationale for the use of magnesium and malic acid." *P J Nutr Med,* vol. 3, pp. 49–59, 1992

CHAPTER 10

1. "Nowhere to hide: persistent toxic chemicals in the U.S. food supply." Pesticide Action Network North America (PANNA)

and Commonweal. 2000. www.panna.org, (415) 981–1771; www.commonweal.org.

2. Centers for Disease Control and Prevention press conference, Atlanta, GA, March 21, 2001

3. "GAO finds that USDA, EPA have neglected pledge to cut pesticide use." U.S. General Accounting Office, U.S. Newswire, September 27, 2001, available at www.gao.gov

4. Kreutzer R et al., "Prevalence of people reporting sensitivities to chemicals in a population-based survey." *Am J Epidemiol,* vol. 150, no. 1, pp. 1–12, 1999

5. "Everyday carcinogens: stopping cancer before it starts." Workshop on Primary Cancer Prevention. McMaster University, Hamilton, Ontario, Canada. March 26–27, 1999

6. Deborah Baker, personal communication. Dr. Baker shares her mercury research at www.y2khealthanddetox.com

7. Goering PL et al., "Toxicity assessment of mercury vapor from dental amalgams." *Fundam Appl Toxicol,* vol. 19, no. 3, pp. 319–329, 1992

8. Halbach S, "Amalgam tooth fillings and man's mercury burden. Review." *Hum Exp Toxicol,* vol. 13, no. 7, pp. 496–501, 1994

9. Lorscheider FL et al., "Mercury exposure from 'silver' tooth fillings: emerging evidence questions a traditional dental paradigm." *FASEB J,* vol. 9, no. 7, pp. 504–508, 1995

10. Arenholt-Bindslev D, Larsen AH, "Mercury levels and discharge in waste water from dental clinics." *Water Air Soil Pollut,* vol. 86, nos. 1–4, pp. 93–99, 1996

11. Drasch G et al., "Comparison of the body burden of the population of Leipzig and Munich with the heavy metals cadmium, lead and mercury—a study of human organ samples." *Gesundheitswesen,* vol. 56, no. 5, pp. 263–267, 1994

12. Liu XY, Jin TY, Nordberg GF, "Increased urinary calcium and magnesium excretion in rats injected with mercuric chloride." *Pharmacol Toxicol,* vol. 68, no. 4, pp. 254–259, 1991

13. Durlach J, "Diverse applications of magnesium therapy. Part five, chapter 1, section B. Handbook of metal-ligand interactions in biological fluids," in *Bioinorganic Medicine,* vol. 2, Marcel Dekker, New York, 1995

14. Kedryna T et al., "Effect of environmental fluorides on key biochemical processes in humans." *Folia Med Cracov,* vol. 34, no. 1–4, pp. 49–57, 1993

15. Semczuk M, Semczuk-Sikora A, "New data on toxic metal intoxication (Cd, Pb, and Hg in particular) and Mg status during pregnancy. Review." *Med Sci Monit,* vol. 7, no. 2, pp. 332–340, 2001

16. Ibid.

17. Durlach J et al., "Magnesium: a competitive inhibitor of lead and cadmium. Ultrastructure studies of the human amniotic epithelial cell." *Magnesium Res,* vol. 3, pp. 31–36, 1990

18. Soldatovic D et al., "Contribution to interaction between magnesium and toxic metals: the effect of prolonged cadmium intoxication on magnesium metabolism in rabbits." *Magnes Res,* vol. 11, no. 4, pp. 283–288, 1998

19. Allen VG, "Influence of aluminum on magnesium metabolism." In: Altura BM, Durlach J, Seelig MS, eds., *Magnesium in Cellular Processes and Medicine.* Krager, Basel, pp. 50–66, 1987

20. Rogers S, *The EI Syndrome: A Rx for Environmental Illness.* Rev. ed. SK Publishing, Sarasota, FL, 1995.

21. Seelig M, "Consequences of magnesium deficiency on the enhancement of stress reactions; preventive and therapeutic implications (a review)." *J Am Coll Nutr,* vol. 13, no. 5, pp. 429–446, 1994

22. *Physicians' Desk Reference*

23. Gurkan F et al., "Intravenous magnesium sulphate in the management of moderate to severe acute asthmatic children nonresponding to conventional therapy." *Eur J Emerg Medicine,* vol. 6, no. 3, pp. 201–205, 1999

24. Ciarallo L et al., "Intravenous magnesium therapy for moderate to severe pediatric asthma: results of a randomized, placebo-controlled trial." *J Pediatr,* vol. 129, pp. 809–814, 1996

25. Dominguez LJ et al., "Bronchial reactivity and intracellular magnesium: a possible mechanism for the bronchodilating effects of magnesium in asthma." *Clin Sci (Colch),* vol. 95, no. 2, pp. 137–142, 1998

26. Britton J, "Dietary magnesium, lung function, wheezing and airway hyperreactivity in a random population sample." *Lancet,* vol. 344, pp. 357–362, 1994

CHAPTER 11

1. Barbagallo M et al., "Cellular ionic alterations with age: relation to hypertension and diabetes." *J Am Geriatr Soc,* vol. 48, no. 9, pp. 1111-1116, 2000

2. Barbagallo M, "Diabetes mellitus, hypertension and ageing: the ionic hypothesis of ageing and cardiovascular-metabolic diseases." *Diabetes Metab,* vol. 23, no. 4, pp. 281–294, 1997

3. Hartwig A, "Role of magnesium in genomic stability." *Mutat Research,* vol. 18, no. 475 (1–2), pp. 113–121, 2001

4. Worwag M et al., "Prevalence of magnesium and zinc deficiencies in nursing home residents in Germany." *Magnes Res,* vol. 12, no. 3, pp. 181–189, 1999

5. Paolisso G et al., "Mean arterial blood pressure and serum levels of the molar ratio of insulin-like growth factor-1 to its binding protein-3 in centenarians." *J Hypertens,* vol. 17, pp. 67–73, 1999

6. Li W et al., "Antioxidants prevent elevation in [Ca(2+)](i) induced by low extracellular magnesium in cultured canine cerebral vascular smooth muscle cells: possible relationship to Mg(2+) deficiency-induced vasospasm and stroke." *Brain Res Bull,* vol. 52, no. 2, pp. 151–154, 2000

7. Hartwig A, "Role of magnesium in genomic stability." *Mutat Research,* vol. 18, no. 475 (1–2), pp. 113–121, 2001

8. Blaylock RL, *Excitotoxins: The Taste That Kills,* Health Press, Sante Fe, NM, 1997

9. Nelson L, "Pesticides and Parkinson's Disease." American Academy of Neurology's 52nd Annual Meeting, San Diego, CA, April 29–May 6, 2000

10. Blaylock RL, *Excitotoxins: The Taste That Kills,* Health Press, Sante Fe, NM, 1997

11. Rondeau V et al., "Aluminum in drinking water and cognitive decline in elderly subjects: the Paquid cohort." *Am J Epidemiol,* vol. 154, no. 3, pp. 288–290, 2001

12. Rondeau V et al., "Relation between aluminum concentrations in drinking water and Alzheimer's disease: an 8-year follow-up study." *Am J Epidemiol,* vol. 152, pp. 59–66, 2000

13. Andrasi E et al., "Disturbances of magnesium concentrations in various brain areas in Alzheimer's disease." *Magnes Res,* vol. 13, no. 3, pp. 189–196, 2000

14. Yasui M et al., "Calcium, magnesium and aluminum concentrations in Parkinson's disease." *Neurotoxicology,* vol. 13, no. 3, pp. 593–600, 1992
15. Blaylock RL, *Excitotoxins: The Taste That Kills,* Health Press, Sante Fe, NM, 1997
16. Durlach J, "Diverse applications of magnesium therapy. Part five, chapter 1, section B. Handbook of metal-ligand interactions in biological fluids." In: *Bioinorganic Medicine,* vol. 2, Marcel Dekker, New York, 1995
17. Blaylock RL, *Excitotoxins: The Taste That Kills,* Health Press, Sante Fe, NM, 1997
18. Durlach J et al., "Magnesium and ageing. II. Clinical data: aetiological mechanisms and pathophysiological consequences of magnesium deficit in the elderly." *Magnes Res,* vol. 6, no. 4, pp. 379–394, 1993

CHAPTER 12
1. Seelig MS, "The requirement of magnesium by the normal adult." *Am J Clin Nutr,* vol. 14, pp. 342–390, 1964
2. Seelig MS, "Magnesium requirements in human nutrition." *Magnes Bull,* vol. 3 (1A), pp. 26–47, 1981
3. Franz KB, "Magnesium intake during pregnancy." *Magnesium,* vol. 6, pp. 18–27, 1987
4. Seelig MS, "The requirement of magnesium by the normal adult." *Am J Clin Nutr,* vol. 14, pp. 342–390, 1964
5. Seelig MS, "Magnesium requirements in human nutrition." *Magnes Bull,* vol. 3 (1A), pp. 26–47, 1981
6. Glei M et al., "Magnesium content of foodstuffs and beverages and magnesium intake of adults in Germany." *Magnes Bull,* vol. 17, pp. 22–28, 1995
7. Cashman KD et al., "Optimal nutrition: calcium, magnesium, and phosphorous." *Proc Nutr Soc,* vol. 58, pp. 477–487, 1999
8. Mircetic RN, Dodig S, Raos M, Petres B, Cepelak I, "Magnesium concentration in plasma, leukocytes and urine of children with intermittent asthma." *Clin Chim Acta,* vol. 312, nos. 1–2, pp. 197–203, 2001
9. Ryzen E et al., "Parenteral magnesium tolerance testing in the evaluation of magnesium deficiency." *Magnesium,* vol. 4, pp. 137–147, 1985

10. Burton Altura, personal communication, November 2001

11. Altura BM, Altura BT, "Role of magnesium in patho-physiological processes and the clinical utility of magnesium ion selective electrodes." *Scand J Clin Lab Invest Suppl,* vol. 224, pp. 211–234, 1996

12. Altura BT, Altura BM, "A method for distinguishing ionized, complexed and protein-bound Mg in normal and diseased subjects." *Scand J Clin Lab Invest Suppl,* vol. 217, pp. 83–87, 1994

13. Altura BT et al., "Comparative findings on serum IMg2+ of normal and diseased human subjects with the NOVA and KONE ISE's for Mg2+." *Scand J Clin Lab Invest Suppl,* vol. 217, pp. 77–81, 1994

14. Altura BT et al., "Characterization of a new ion selective electrode for ionized magnesium in whole blood, plasma, serum, and aqueous samples." *Scand J Clin Lab Invest Suppl,* vol. 217, pp. 21–36, 1994

15. Altura BT et al., "A new method for the rapid determination of ionized Mg2+ in whole blood, serum and plasma." *Methods and Findings in Exp Clin Pharmacol,* vol. 4, pp. 297–304, 1992

16. Altura BT, Altura BM, "Measurement of ionized magnesium in whole blood, plasma and serum with a new ion-selective electrode in healthy and diseased human subjects." *Magnes Trace Elem,* vol. 10, nos. 2–4, pp. 90–98, 1991–1992

17. Altura BT, Altura BM, "A method for distinguishing ionized, complexed and protein-bound Mg in normal and diseased subjects." *Scand J Clin Lab Invest Suppl,* vol. 217, pp. 83–87, 1994

18. Altura BM, Altura BT, "Role of magnesium in patho-physiological processes and the clinical utility of magnesium ion selective electrodes." *Scand J Clin Lab Invest Suppl,* vol. 224, pp. 211–234, 1996

19. Ibid.

20. Personal communication with Burton Altura, November 2001

21. Altura BT et al., "Clinical studies with the NOVA ISE for IMg2+." *Scand J Clin Lab Invest Suppl,* vol. 217, pp. 53–67, 1994

22. Marcus JC, Altura BT, Altura BM, "Serum ionized magnesium in post-traumatic headaches." *J Pediatr,* vol. 139, no. 3, pp. 459–462, 2001

23. Muneyvirci-Delale O et al., "Divalent cations in women with PCOS: implications for cardiovascular disease." *Gynecol Endocrinol,* vol. 3, pp. 198–201, 2001

24. Marcus JC et al., "Serum ionized magnesium in premature and term infants." *Pediatr Neurol*, vol. 4, pp. 311–314, 1998
25. Scott VL et al., "Ionized hypomagnesemia in patients undergoing orthotopic liver transplantation: a complication of citrate intoxication." *Liver Transpl Surg*, vol. 2, no. 5, pp. 343–347, 1996
26. Altura BT et al., "Low levels of serum ionized magnesium are found in patients early after stroke which result in rapid elevation in cytosolic free calcium and spasm in cerebral vascular muscle cells." *Neurosci Lett*, vol. 230, no. 1, pp. 37–40, 1997
27. Handwerker SM, Altura BT, Altura BM, "Serum ionized magnesium and other electrolytes in the antenatal period of human pregnancy." *J Am Coll Nutr*, vol. 15, no. 1, pp. 36–43, 1996
28. Memon ZI et al., "Predictive value of serum ionized but not total magnesium levels in head injuries." *Scand J Clin Lab Invest*, vol. 55, no. 8, pp. 671–677, 1995
29. Handwerker SM, Altura BT, Altura BM, "Ionized serum magnesium and potassium levels in pregnant women with preeclampsia and eclampsia." *J Reprod Medicine*, vol. 40, no. 3, pp. 201–208, 1995
30. Drs. Bella and Burton Altura, State University of New York, Health Science Center at Brooklyn, New York
31. Durlach J, Bac P, Bara M, Guiet-Bara A, "Cardiovasoprotective foods and nutrients: possible importance of magnesium intake." *Magnes Res*, vol. 12, no. 1, pp. 57–61, 1999
32. Murray M, *Encyclopedia of Nutritional Supplements,* Prima Publishing, Rocklin, CA, 1996
33. Wood M, *Seven Herbs: Plants as Teachers,* North Atlantic Books, Berkeley, CA, 1987
34. Weed S, *Healing Wise: The Wise Woman Herbal,* Ash Tree Publishing, Woodstock, NY, 1989
35. Duke JA, *The Green Pharmacy,* St. Martin's Press, New York, 1998
36. Chevallier A, *The Encyclopedia of Medicinal Plants,* DK Publishing, New York, 1996
37. Marx A et al., "Magnesium in drinking water and ischemic heart disease." *Epididemiol Rev*, vol. 19, pp. 258–272, 1997

38. Von Wiesenberger A, *The Pocket Guide to Bottled Water*, Contemporary Books, Chicago, 1991

CHAPTER 13

1. Durlach J, *Magnesium in Clinical Practice*, Libbey, London, 1988.
2. Fehlinger R, "Therapy with magnesium salts in neurological diseases." *Magnes Bull*, vol. 12, pp. 35–42, 1990
3. Ducroix T, "L'enfant spasmophile—Aspects diagnostiques et therapeutiques." *Magnes Bull*, vol. 1, pp. 9–15, 1984
4. Seelig MS, "Athletic stress, performance and magnesium in consequences of magnesium deficiency on the enhancement of stress reactions; preventive and therapeutic implications: a review." *J Am Coll Nutr*, vol. 13, no. 5, pp. 429–446, 1994
5. Seelig MS, "Magnesium requirements in human nutrition." *Magnes Bull*, vol. 3 (1A), pp. 26–47, 1981
6. Johnson S, "The multifaceted and widespread pathology of magnesium deficiency." *Med Hypotheses*, vol. 56, no. 2, pp. 163–170, 2001
7. Rude RK et al., "Low serum concentrations of 1,25-dihydroxyvitamin D in human magnesium deficiency." *J Clin Endocrinol Metab*, vol. 61, pp. 833–940, 1985
8. Fuss M et al., "Correction of low circulating levels of 1,25-dihydroxyvitamin D by 25-hydroxyvitamin D during reversal of hypomagnesaemia." *Clinical Endocrinol Oxf*, vol. 31, pp. 31–38, 1989
9. Manuel y Keenoy B, Moorkens G, Vertommen J, Noe M, Neve J, De Leeuw I, "Magnesium status and parameters of the oxidant-antioxidant balance in patients with chronic fatigue: effects of supplementation with magnesium." *J Am Coll Nutr*, vol. 19, no. 3, pp. 374–382, 2000
10. Boericke OE, *Pocket Manual of Homeopathic Materia Medica*, 9th ed., Boericke & Runyon, Philadelphia, 1927

Index

attention deficit hyperactivity
disorder (ADHD), 51, 66

back pain, 6, 18, 19, 134
birth control pills, 37, 164, 166
blood clots, 5, 52, 68–69, 84, 92,
101, 102, 103
blood pressure, 3, 96
high, *see* hypertension
blood sugar, 5, 13, 17, 48, 49, 96, 100
low, 66–68
bond density, 139–47
test, 139–40
bone meal, 226–27
bowel disease, 5, 20
bowel obstruction, 226
bowel movements:
loose, 225, 226, 229, 230
regular, 20
brain, 23–24, 27, 52, 119
Alzheimer's disease and,
195–203
damage, 136–38, 213
magnesium and, 63–80
surgery, and magnesium, 76–77,
78
burdock root, 219–20
burns, third-degree, 8

cadmium, 178, 197, 231
calcium, 3, 13, 22, 23, 33, 50, 68,
76, 78, 80, 105, 119, 121, 126,
130, 147, 192, 193, 209
deficiency, 16
and drug interactions in heart
disease, 94, 95
excess, 13, 16, 23, 27, 28, 59, 86,
87, 107, 111, 140, 144, 231
kidney stones and, 147–52
magnesium and, 26–29, 112,
139–52, 221, 231
in mineral water, 221–23
osteoporosis and, 139–47
supplementation with

magnesium, 9, 17, 19, 21, 28,
29, 112, 124, 130, 140–52, 231
cancer, 8, 57, 58, 174
environmental toxins and, 174–76
magnesium and, 58
carbohydrates, 61, 66, 116, 118,
129, 217
cardiac death syndrome, 61–62
cardiovascular metabolic syndrome
(CVMS), 111–12, 113
cells, 21, 27
death, 66
metabolism, 3, 21, 27
cerebral palsy, 7, 136–38
chelated magnesium, 227
chelation therapy, 107–8
chickweed, 220
children, 162, 163, 164, 207, 225, 234
asthma, 184, 186–87, 210
cerebral palsy, 136–38
diabetic, 117–18
magnesium-deficient, 51–52
SIDS, 135–36
chocolate, 127, 148
cholesterol, 20, 61, 81, 88–91, 92,
96, 109, 110, 113, 116, 117
magnesium and, 88–91
LDL vs. HDL, 88–89
chronic fatigue syndrome, 60,
155–70, 172
magnesium and, 155–70
cilantro, 219
cluster headaches, 70–71
coffee, 36, 89, 105, 109, 129, 142,
148, 149
constipation, 5, 20, 134, 199
contraindications to magnesium
therapy, 226
cortisone, 37, 50, 162–64
cramps, 6, 9
leg, 9, 13–14, 16, 49, 53, 55–57,
61, 193, 228, 233–34
menstrual, 7, 15, 20, 26
cystitis, 5

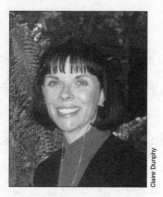

Claire Dunphy

About the Author

CAROLYN DEAN, M.D., N.D., is a medical doctor, naturopathic doctor, activist, environmentalist, acupuncturist, homeopath, herbalist, clinical nutritionist, writer, researcher, and inventor. The focus of her medical practice, from its inception in 1979, was to teach people about natural options and choices to achieve optimum health. In 2002, Dr. Dean and her business partner, Delia Quigley, launched Halo Works organic herbal tinctures and began offering the Body Rejuvenation Cleanse Program in New York. Dr. Dean's Web site is www.carolyndean.com.